SWIMMINGLY

SWIMMINGLY

ADVENTURES
IN WATER

VASSOS ALEXANDER

BLOOMSBURY SPORT
LONDON · OXFORD · NEW YORK · NEW DELHI · SYDNEY

BLOOMSBURY SPORT
Bloomsbury Publishing Plc
50 Bedford Square, London, WC1B 3DP, UK
Bloomsbury Publishing Ireland Limited,
29 Earlsfort Terrace, Dublin 2, D02 AY28, Ireland

First published in Great Britain, 2025

Photography: p. 6 (top left) © @evolutiondrone; p 8 (top) © Alamy Images;
(middle and bottom left) © Getty Images

A catalogue record for this book is available from the British Library

Library of Congress Cataloguing-in-Publication data has been applied for

ISBN: HB: 978-1-399-41459-3; ePUB: 978-1-399-41458-6; ePDF: 978-1-3994-1455-5

2 4 6 8 10 9 7 5 3 1

Typeset in Minion Pro by Deanta Global Publishing Services, Chennai, India
Printed and bound in Great Britain by CPI (Group) UK Ltd, Croydon, CR0 4YY

MIX
Paper | Supporting
responsible forestry
FSC® C013604

To find out more about our authors and books visit www.bloomsbury.com and sign up
for our newsletters

For product safety related questions contact productsafety@bloomsbury.com

CONTENTS

INTRODUCTION

This is a book that was always heading one way, only to change its mind at the last minute. It was meant to be a swim Odyssey across the Channel to Calais, and only made it about as far as the 'Welcome to Dover' sign. All through writing, the plan was to finish on a French beach after a journey of 21 miles and several years. The final chapter was going to be the story of me swimming the Channel. Now the book ends with me conclusively *not swimming the Channel*.

Reader, I promise it wasn't for lack of effort or commitment. And here's the thing. I'm thrilled at how it all worked out. Or rather, how it didn't work out – and we'll get to that. But let's start in Greece.

A bit of this book was born on the island of Euboea in the 1980s. Born of childhood summers spent in the house my grandfather built by the sea. It was a good 20 minutes' drive down several dirt tracks to the nearest village and telephone, so the only thing to do was swim. And I grew to love it there. The bungalow, the stony beach, the clear, blue Med with the mainland on the horizon. The sea became our playground, drifting, diving and dodging the odd jellyfish. The waves whispered secrets of adventure, while every splash of water against skin was a call to freedom. Swimming seemed to have a language all its own. I learned to listen to the rhythm of the tides, the mysterious life beneath the surface, the stories the ocean had to tell.

Later Papou bought a speedboat and waterskiing became the main event. Suddenly we were only in the sea because we fell in while learning a new trick. We thought life had become better. We didn't realise what we were missing.

This book was also born on a cross-Channel ferry in the mid-90s. I'd just turned 20 and was driving to Paris with a new girlfriend in an old Peugeot. Caroline, now my wife, was reading about Captain Matthew Webb in the on-board magazine. He was the first person to complete a solo Channel swim, in 1875. It blew my mind that someone could swim these murky, choppy waters wearing nothing but a swimsuit, goggles and cap. The idea of doing so gave me that same shiver of excitement whenever someone suggests biting off more than I can chew. Getting outside your comfort zone, occasionally massively, seems like a great way to suck the most out of life. One day, I thought, one day... And then we reached Paris and I forgot all about it.

Until I spent a night in the Nottingham Holiday Inn in 2013. I'd just completed my first proper endurance event, an Ironman triathlon, and was sweating buckets. Literally, buckets. Sweating so much I had to turn over the soaking mattress, only to discover the sweat had gone right through and it was almost as wet on the other side. Strange, how the body reacts after extreme stress. And while I was sweating, I saw things very vividly, almost as if on hallucinogens. And the thing I saw clearly in Nottingham, was swimming. It had been my first triathlon, and my first organised swim of any kind. I'd been dreading that 2.4-mile swim leg. But to my shock and delight, I adored it. So much so, I was sad when it was time to get out of the wetsuit and onto the bike. And that night in Nottingham, between the sweat-sodden sheets, I heard an echo of the exhilaration of those childhood summers. I remembered how swimming encourages thoughts to drift like clouds, untethered and free. How each stroke becomes a celebration of being alive.

So I joined the Serpentine Swim Club in London's Hyde Park. Surrounded by open water swimmers, I discovered a community bound by shared challenges and triumphs. A unique blend of serenity, adventure and banter. Everyone brought their own journey, and some had already completed the most famous swimming journey of all – that solo crossing between Shakespeare Beach in Kent and Cap Gris Nez near Calais.

Another part of the book was born on a sandy beach on the Isle of Wight after swimming across the Solent. Another in the London 2012 Olympic pool where I was the very first person to race. And another in a bay in Jersey where I met a bona fide Channel legend.

But mainly this book was born over brunch in Borough Market. A general catch up with long-time editor and friend Charlotte. I told her how swimming had become my latest obsession. I thought I was on pretty safe ground, after all I'm the running books guy. And then I looked up and noticed a familiar glint in Charlotte's eye. The glint that usually ends with me gleefully deciding to do something silly and writing about it. Soon I was signing a contract to write a book about swimming the Channel... That's this book, in which I don't swim the Channel. Which will come as a bit of a shock to me.

In the meantime I carried on training and writing until my time came: position three on the Spring tide of 10–15 September 2024. Some of the training was immense. Back-to-back eight-hour swims starting in the middle of the night in the middle of nowhere. Swimming across a bay full of sharks. Practice swim drills punctuating a family holiday in Mauritius. Winter dips in the North Sea. Ice baths at dawn. I loved it all.

I loved the organisation a lot less. There's a ton of form-filling involved in a Channel attempt, and mine were invariably late. One example – the medical which has to be submitted to the Channel Swimming and Piloting Federation, at the very latest, by the end of April. They received mine in August. They were very kind as their patience was tested again and again. Turns out my somewhat haphazard approach to life suits ultra swimming a lot less than it suits endurance running. I once turned up at a trail race without running shoes and ran 62 hilly miles in what were basically gardening shoes. Not recommended, obviously, and yet I find a certain freedom and joy in the slapdash.

So you're not going to read the story of someone swimming solo across the Channel. A combination, since you ask, of poor planning, a gammy shoulder and some very unfortunate weather. But you are going to read the story of someone discovering a sport – a movement even – brimming with welcoming, togetherness and positivity. At the heart of both running and swimming is a massive sense of community.

Along the way we'll swim the length of London via lakes and lidos. We'll swim from town to town along the Thames, and endlessly up and down Bournemouth beachfront. We'll learn the correct form for the front crawl and we'll escape from Alcatraz. We'll meet Olympic champions and Channel legends, as well as a group of (mostly) middle-aged women discovering how swimming can massively improve your day, your week, your life. We'll meet the Edmund Hillary of the oceans and a woman so extraordinary she's had an Oscar-nominated film made about her. As well as an American who went for a swim one day, and saved the world.

Let's begin – of course – in the middle. Specifically the middle of peak Channel training and the middle of San Francisco Bay teeming with sharks. Nothing like the threat of an imminent Great White attack to persuade you to read on...

1

Swimming Alcatraz

I'm terrified. I'm freezing. And also – how can this be?! – I'm a bit bored.

Freezing, because I'm on an open, inflatable boat in very rough seas wearing nothing but shorts and a swim cap. Bored, because I'm midway through an infernal 75-minute wait for a vast tanker to make an appearance before I can start swimming. And terrified, because of the sharks.

This is the famous Alcatraz Swim, organised every July by a swimming club in San Francisco. There are around 30 of us signed up for the swim of around two miles and we're aboard three small boats. We should all have been in the water an hour ago, but for the delay caused by the tanker. The US Coast Guard understandably wants it to have rolled through before we're allowed to start. I know from our pilot that the tanker – or 'deep draft vessel' as he calls it – is coming from the west, under Golden Gate Bridge, but frustratingly there's still no sign of it. Meanwhile I'm allowing my fears to spiral.

The event has a regular photographer who's sitting directly in front of me. She says she's never seen it this rough for the swim. White horses are everywhere. The pilot chimes in that he's never seen the local fishing fleet so close to Alcatraz Island; there are several dozen boats all within a few hundred metres of the former prison.

Two thoughts are whirling around in my head. First, is it safe to swim in this much swell? The organisers are on boat one so I can't ask them. We've been graded by our estimated finish time and I must have over-lied because I've ended up on boat three with the quickest swimmers, who all look like they've come straight from the US National Championships. I booked this so long ago I can't honestly remember what time I said I could swim two miles in, but I definitely exaggerated massively to make sure I was allowed to come along. The website said only very experienced open water swimmers could apply. It means I'll be one of the last in the sea, which looks like it's getting rougher by the minute.

Also, as the pilot says, there are fishing boats near Alcatraz 'for the first time ever'. If that's where the fishing fleet has congregated, then that's obviously where the fish are. And if that's where the fish are, that's also surely where the great whites are, too. This event has never yet lost a swimmer to a shark attack, but with unprecedented waves and those damn fishing boats so close, these do seem like ideal conditions to buck that trend. Only a year ago, a local tech entrepreneur was attacked and pulled under the water by sharks just a short distance north of here.

Alcatraz was originally built as a naval defence fort and was turned into a prison early in the 20th century. It was immediately branded 'inescapable' because of its isolation, steep cliffs and the swift, cold currents that surround it. Alcatraz was home to some of the most notorious convicts of all time including gangsters Al Capone, Mickey Cohen and George 'Machine Gun' Kelly.

San Francisco residents slept soundly in their beds knowing it was impossible to escape from 'The Rock'. Only a foolhardy few gave it a try. Most famously, in June 1962 a particularly inventive trio – Frank Morris, and brothers John and Clarence Anglin – escaped through an air duct which they'd chiselled loose over months using spoons, disguising the noise by playing the accordion. They left plaster moulds of their heads in their beds to fool the guards, and set off to sea on a life raft made of raincoats donated by fellow convicts. They were never heard from again, with the FBI concluding they drowned within a few hundred metres of the island. Despite 36 attempts, nobody successfully escaped from Alcatraz and now I'm beginning to understand why. This is a tough two miles to swim.

Weirdly, the swimmers behind me on the boat don't seem remotely worried. A mixture of locals and tourists in town especially for the swim, they're discussing how come US workers typically receive just two weeks' annual holiday and the best ways of using them. A woman behind me suddenly announces that her dad was an Olympian. A professional swim instructor on board chimes in that he coached a member of the USA Olympic water polo team who at that exact moment is competing against Greece at the Paris Games (USA won and the swimmer in question scored; I looked it up later).

I'd usually join in the banter, but I couldn't be less in the mood. My teeth are the only part of me wanting to chatter. I'm successfully persuading myself there's a reasonable chance that I might die in the next hour. I'm going so far as to imagine what it's like to be eaten by a shark. The adrenaline will probably mask the pain, I figure, and at least it'll be quick. I come to the conclusion that it's far better to be eaten than to drown. And it'll make a dramatic story for the funeral.

Most of the others are wearing wetsuits and I'm one of very few 'skins'. Would a shark go for a wetsuit swimmer first on account of looking more like a seal? Or is that not a thing? How come nobody else is panicking? If we were still on dry land, I'd seriously consider pulling out. I may yet. And by the way, why *aren't* we still on dry land? Why do we have to wait on the boats? By now even my legs are turning blue and I'm beginning to feel seasick.

I resort to breathing exercises and mantras to calm the nerves and pass the time. Eventually the 'deep draft vessel' appears under the famous red suspension bridge. It's big, but disappointingly not massive. After all this sitting around I'd been hoping for something awesome. I once caught sight of the world's biggest container ship, Barzan, on its way to Southampton: 400 metres long with almost 20,000 containers on board. Now seeing THAT up close might have been worth an hour's freezing wait.

The ship goes past and three things happen simultaneously. The rib we're on is caught side-on by a huge wave, sending a jet of sea water up my nose. At the exact same time, seemingly connected to the nasal flush, our pilot's radio buzzes into life. And from the side of one of the other boats, a swimmer jumps into the water.

The first boat, a tourist vessel painted yellow to look like some kind of aquatic New York taxi, swiftly disgorges its cargo of about a dozen swimmers and the sea is full of brightly coloured tow floats. Next they start diving off the second boat, another inflatable, one after the other, until the pilot is the only person on board. And suddenly it's our turn. We've been given numbers, the order we're meant to start in, but my mind goes blank and I can't remember mine. It was written in marker pen on my hand and the sea's long since erased it. A woman jumps in, a bloke accidentally elbows me in the temple as he follows, and before I know it, I'm thinking sod it and joining them in the intimidating water.

Right, so this is happening. Better start swimming.

The advice is to aim for the Fontana Towers in San Francisco's Fisherman's Wharf district and allow the current to take you to the finish at the Yacht Club. Trouble is, I can't make out any landmarks through the waves and the fog in my goggles. Can't even see any fellow swimmers to follow. Orange tow floats have disappeared behind white horses. The waves are piling in from the west, from our right, and the current is coming from the east, pushing us back towards the Golden Gate Bridge. I'm way out of my depth. Literally and figuratively.

All the ingredients are there for panic and I'm shocked to discover that it never arrives. I may not be able to see the Fontana Towers, but obviously I can see San Francisco, so I just swim that way. If I end up too far to the left, I can always swim west with the current along the shore until I reach the Yacht Club. If I end up too far to the right, it's game over as the current is too strong to swim against. One of the boats would have to pick me up.

The water is cold but not freezing. I'm pretty good at this by now and my skin thermometer guesstimates the temperature in the Bay to be around 15 degrees Celsius. Perfect too, for my six-hour Channel qualifier, which I've still not managed. But that's a problem for tomorrow. Right now I've got massive waves coming at me from my right, making it hard to breathe on that side. I persist, because that's the side where the Golden Gate Bridge is and I definitely want to keep seeing that.

I end up drinking quite a lot of San Francisco Bay. Every few seconds, along with the waves, the fact hits me that I'm swimming above hundreds of sharks. At the best of times it's easy to let your mind wander to what's lurking in the depths. Yet somehow, when I know for a fact that there are beasties below, I relax. It's like that moment when, caught in a rainstorm without an umbrella, you abandon your futile efforts to stay dry and accept getting soaked through. Something inside unclenches. I realise there's nothing I can do about the sharks and calmly (relatively calmly) focus on my stroke.

I've rarely swum in such large swell, and it takes some getting used to. I soon abandon my plan to enjoy looking up at the Golden Gate Bridge, and breathe only to the left. The amount of sea water I ingest instantly drops from loads to hardly any.

Other issues do persist. With the waves towering above, I largely don't have a clue where I am. A couple of times I pause to get my bearings and realise I've somehow started swimming in exactly the wrong direction, back towards Alcatraz. I hastily turn around and hope none of the rescue boats have noticed. It would be highly embarrassing to be picked up for swimming backwards.

After a few minutes, I remember to start my watch. Garmins find it notoriously difficult to accurately track open water swims – most of the time they're underwater – but they do manage to get the map largely right. And I realise the map of this swim will look fantastic: a red line arcing from Alcatraz Island to San Francisco Yacht Club. Got to swim it first though.

Occasionally, the breathing stroke happens when I'm at the top of a wave and plunging back down feels a little like a funfair ride. There's also the exciting way time becomes elastic while you're swimming. The first few minutes seem to stretch into hours, before speeding up again so that the minutes go by in seconds. My watch vibrates on my wrist every 500 metres and the first vibration takes so long to come I fear the watch is broken.

By the time I do feel the reassuring buzz on my wrist, I've settled into a rhythm. I've been training hard with the aim of one day becoming what swim coaches call 'a passenger in my own stroke'. Today it happens without my noticing. Left arm, right arm, left arm, breathe... Left arm, right arm, left arm, breathe... The world contracts to become a dance with the waves. The stroke, the effort, the fresh feel of water against skin, the sound of the breath. Awareness of form and technique soon gives way to a sense of flow and tranquillity. In no time at all, the Garmin vibrates for a second time and I barely notice. And then a third, fourth, fifth. And suddenly the Yacht Club appears a few hundred metres in front of me.

The swell has reduced significantly so close to the shore. I can now see other swimmers' tow floats heading towards the small sandy beach. I put in a sprint finish and soon regret it. Because before I know it – with a twinge of disappointment – the swim is over.

First things first, I dutifully check in with the marshal on the beach; everybody has to, so they know we're not lost at sea. And then I'm slightly at a loss on shore. Most swimmers are being met by family and friends who've brought clothes and transport. I'm in the minority who are getting back on the boats for a lift back to Fisherman's Wharf. There's a party mood on the beach, but I'm too chilly to join in. I also don't know anybody, having been too terrified to join in the pre-swim banter. They were bonding while I was having a private pantomime panic. I'm shivering now and need to get dressed, but my clothes are in a bag on the boat where I left them.

I realise I felt warmer in the sea than out of it, so I wait submerged in the shallows until the call comes to swim out to one of the boats, the one that looks like a New York taxi. Several people are already on board, including the swimmers who didn't make it to the beach and had to be rescued.

I dress as we potter back along the shore and contemplate the swim. In retrospect, I'm a little embarrassed about how scared I'd been. But I wouldn't swap it. Doesn't matter if the terror had any concrete basis – the fact is I genuinely feared for my life. And like the free climber Alex Honnold says, it's important to feel in mortal danger occasionally, if only to make the rest of life seem less stressful. You can hardly obsess about, say, losing your phone, if you've recently been an inch from death on the sheer face of El Capitan 1000 metres above the ground in Yosemite National Park.

My wife and kids are waiting for me on Pier 39, waving enthusiastically as the boat pulls in. They've just had an adventure of their own – a first ride in one of San Francisco's fabulous driverless taxis. You order on the app, unlock via Bluetooth and away you go. We take one back to the hotel.

Seeing the wheel turn all by itself is strange for all of 30 seconds, before feeling so normal that cars with drivers start to look old-fashioned.

Caroline asks what the swim was like. Fine, I say. Great! Clearly I'll never admit how terrified I'd been. How I somehow managed to persuade myself that I was about to be eaten. But secretly I'm delighted by all of it. You want a swim like Alcatraz to feel somewhat heroic and, whisper it quietly, this really did.

2

Swimming Solent

It's Tuesday evening, it's raining and I'm running slightly too quickly for comfort in London's Richmond Park. This is standard Tuesday evening fare, the weekly Barnes Runners club run. I'm chatting to a pal, Sam, and he's trundling up the hill at a pace which makes speaking extremely difficult. I'm doing that thing where you ask open questions to make the other person do most of the talking. I just need to concentrate on breathing and trying to keep up. 'Tell me about your childhood, Sam.' 'What do you think of the upcoming US elections?' 'Where are some of your favourite places to go on holiday?'

He finishes a story about how he once just missed out on the GB Olympic rowing team and I'm forced to find another topic to keep him chatting. I know that Sam's just bought a cottage on the Isle of Wight and steer the conversation that way. I happily tune out as he harps on about how much he loves it there. Then he stops talking abruptly and I realise, to my dismay, that he's waiting for me to answer a question. I replay the last few seconds in my head and he seems to have been asking if I fancy swimming to the Isle of Wight with him.

That's obviously wrong. Nobody swims to the Isle of Wight. I've been several times on the ferry and even that takes ages. And it's one of the busiest shipping lanes in the world. I must have misheard. He must've been saying something like, 'Do you fancy staying on the Isle of Wight with me and let's go swimming while we're there.' We have daughters the same age and a few days together on the island sounds fantastic. 'Thanks Sam. Yes, I'd love to.' 'Great,' he says, 'I'll let you know.' And then he speeds up again making any further conversation, and indeed any more running together, impossible. The last I see of Sam that evening he's disappearing off up the hill towards the ballet school in the centre of the park. I gratefully slow down and look forward to a formal invitation to stay at Sam's holiday place.

The following day an email arrives from someone called Paul Parrish. He's the fundraising and marketing director for Aspire, a charity which organises swimming events and he's thrilled to hear I'll be joining Sam and two other nutters attempting to swim the three miles from Stokes Bay near Portsmouth to Ryde Sands on the Isle of Wight. Wetsuits optional. This is way before I have any inclination to do any serious swimming. I am still chasing running goals. So I call Paul with the intention of wriggling out of it, but am instantly swept along by his enthusiasm:

'I've got this thing about open water swimming. I understand the fear, because it is a hostile environment. I understand how frightening these things are, but also how goddam good you feel afterwards. So to me, it's the perfect fundraiser. You do something that's good for other people, but you also feel brilliant yourself. And it's a springboard, isn't it, to something else? To a better version of you.

'I happened to join Aspire at the same time I was looking to swim the Channel solo. They were the only charity in the country that were doing anything around open water swimming. They already had a toe in the water, as it were. So I arrived and we had a guy called Andrew, who was really good at it and who was also a fantastic organiser, and what started as a vanity project just got bigger and bigger, as we both kept identifying other swims, and putting more and more effort into it.

'We started getting a bit of a following as there was simultaneously a huge surge in open water swimming. We just happened to be the beneficiaries, in the right place at the right time, but we had the knowledge, so it's done really well for us. I'm meant to be in front of a spreadsheet, but actually I've spent most of my life on boats, helping people go across the Channel or the Solent, and I love it.'

So suddenly it became a thing. I signed up for my first swim of any significance and couldn't stop telling people about it. Not that I did any training. I was still determined to run a road marathon PB and all my athletic energies were directed towards an (ultimately disappointing) Amsterdam marathon, but a month before we were due to muster in Portsmouth, I found out I needed to have a two-hour swim under my belt and it needed to be witnessed. As luck would have it, I happened to be on my way to the South of France at the time with my mate Tom. Perfect!

It was a choppy afternoon in the warm, blue waters of the Med when I essentially doubled the distance of my previous longest swim. I swam up and down the same bay so Tom, who was happily reading a novel in the sun, could keep half an eye on me and verify the swim. I was feeling sluggish and felt tired within five minutes. Then I was stung by a jellyfish and briefly considered abandoning. This, I thought to myself, might prove tough.

But it wasn't tough at all, it was wonderful. Just me and the waves and the currents and the blue sky above – and the occasional painful jellyfish sting. I couldn't believe it when I noticed Tom waving at me from the beach and checked my watch. I'd been swimming for over two hours and it had gone by in a flash. With my face buried underwater, time had twisted into nothing. I began impatiently counting the days to the Isle of Wight swim.

I met Paul in person on the morning of the swim. He has an impressive list of ultra-swimming achievements under his belt, especially for someone who couldn't swim at all until early middle age:

'My father's disabled, we never went swimming as kids, so I was in my late 30s and I wanted to do a triathlon. I'd been very unfit and just starting in recovery from alcohol addiction. I wanted to do a triathlon, but couldn't swim. So I started going down to a pool and looking at what people did... I learned the rudiments from doing that. Literally from watching others.

'And then I got into endurance triathlon, which meant that I was starting to go really long distances. I made sure I hit every swimming session with the triathlon club and the swimming started to become the strongest part of my triathlon.

'I ended up doing a Triple Ironman and the 7.2-mile swim was the bit that I enjoyed most. I thought, okay, there's something in this for me. And then I looked at the Arch to Arc and thought I'd love to do that.'

A quick explanation of the Arch to Arc: it's shorthand for Marble Arch to Arc de Triomphe. It's the toughest triathlon on the planet and one of the toughest endurance events of any kind. You start in London, under Marble Arch. You then run 87 miles to Dover, swim the Channel and cycle to the Champs-Élysées in Paris to finish under the Arc de Triomphe. This is the brainchild of a man called Edgar Ette who, in 2001, devised and completed the challenge. He then formed the company Enduroman to help others follow in his footsteps. Thousands have now attempted an Arch to Arc and 52 have succeeded, including Paul, Enduroman number 20, who completed it in 85 hours after two years of solid training:

'When I entered, I had two years to basically get myself up to Channel swimming fit. I'd heard of people who had managed to do this, although most people told me you had to be from a swim background. And I put everything into it. For two years of my life, I just immersed myself in it. I was very selfish in that respect.

'I was also frightened. I would have panic attacks in open water, but I just kept plugging away, learning to control my own head. Learning how to just stop, look around. Understanding that my brain is the strongest muscle in my body. If you run or cycle, you can stop, have a chat, take some food on, but swimming, you are always immersed in a hostile environment that your brain can tell you is not a good place to be.

'And you're cold and there's stuff in there. There's jellyfish. Anything that touches me in the water, it freaks me out. I'm like, "Whoa! Hey, what's that doing there?"

'The Channel, 10 hours of it were in darkness. I told my crew not to tell me where I was, how long I've been in, anything like that. And you've got no sensory reference whatsoever in the water, especially at night, apart from a boat next to you.

'After God knows how many hours I remember coming up. I could hear industrial machinery. I thought the whole thing had gone wrong. I thought I was off the coast of Calais, which was a really bad sign. I was actually off the coast of rural France. It was a kilometre away from the Cap – Cap Gris-Nez, the bit of France all Channel swimmers are aiming for.

'There was a moment when my right hand touched sand. I will never forget that moment, because I didn't know what was going on. By then I was really out of it. I touched sand on my right hand, it was like, oh my god, what is that? And only when your left hand touches sand, the penny drops. Holy shit! This is it! Amazing feeling. And there's not a day when I don't think about it, even now, and it's been coming up for a decade.'

I can't imagine a more inspirational way to begin my first proper swim. There are four of us, each with a kayaker to guide us across. As we wade in from the beach, I'm happily chatting to the friendly young man assigned to me, part of me looking forward to getting to know him much better in the coming hours. Of course that won't happen, I soon realise, as I'm head down in the choppy Solent.

I'm hoping I won't finish last and force the others to wait for me on the Isle of Wight. We're due to return together in a speedboat once the final swimmer has made the crossing. I don't want that to be me and – happily – it isn't.

I start swimming like a man possessed and soon find myself a long way clear of the others, even Sam. Fortified by my early speed, I settle into a happy rhythm and soon fall into another meditation-like trance. Just the stroke and the breath, the water and the waves.

A couple of memories from that swim: a giant jellyfish, disturbingly close by, with tentacles as long as my shin; the sharp underwater taste of the diesel from the Isle of Wight ferry. Pausing at one point, I look up to see the vast bulk of a container ship. From a duck's perspective, it's the size of a country. I have my first sense of making a journey by water under my own steam and I just feel so lucky to be doing what I am doing.

'About 15 minutes left,' says the kayaker as a sandy beach appears in the near distance. I'm having all the fun and I don't want this swim to end. Fortunately, it's a long 15 minutes, because the tide turns against us. I treasure every moment. I'm the first to arrive and euphoric when I emerge from the sea, but simultaneously gutted, because I want to carry on swimming. I practically 'need' to carry on.

I immediately beg the kayaker to escort me back to Portsmouth. I figure if we leave now, the others will arrive back on the boat at around the same time as us. It's a hard no from the kayaker. He's been itching to stretch his arms and return at full speed. I offer him money. Still no. More money. Nope. Now a ridiculous amount of cash for what will be around 90 minutes' work. Another no and he sets off for home before I can embarrass myself any further.

Which is when I realise that open water swimming may have me hooked.

3

Swimming Downhill I

Why do they call it trial and error? It's a pretty pessimistic name for it. Why not trial and success? But then I find out.

Try, error. Try, error. Try, error.

I'm in a swimming pool underneath a skyscraper in the city of London, attempting something called 'basic extension'. It's very frustrating. With an extra layer of feeling like you're drowning.

Try, error. Try, error. Try, error. Drowning in frustration. Frustratedly drowning.

This is the first of what will become many drills designed to give me the perfect swim stroke for my assault on the Channel. The fact it's called 'basic' makes me feel even worse about my total inability to master it. Here's what you do. Lie in the water on one side, kicking constantly with your feet to stay afloat. One arm lives glued to your side, the other is straight out in front of your chin. You're travelling so slowly the motion is barely perceptible. Every few seconds you tilt your head to breathe, only to mistime it and end up with a lungful of chlorinated water. Try, error. Try, error.

This all started with the phrase 'You've got to go and see Ray!' I was hearing it everywhere, from everyone. Like when you decide to buy a Renault Clio having never really noticed the Renault Clio exists. You're suddenly stunned by how many

20

Renault Clios there are on the road. Frequency illusion, they call it. Ray is the swim-specific version of the Renault Clio. You've never heard of Ray. Why would you have? Then you tell people you're planning to swim the Channel and everyone everywhere chips in with, 'You've got to go and see Ray!' I'm lucky in that the early starts required by my job as sports presenter on the *Chris Evans Breakfast Show* on Virgin Radio give me a fair amount of flexibility during the day. So I go and see Ray.

Ray Gibbs is one the world's great swimming teachers. He only took up swimming in his mid-20s when he began competing in triathlons. A Channel relay in 1992 began his love of open water swimming. Starting from scratch and frustrated by the lack of clear information on how to become a distance swimmer, he watched the technique of the talented ex-GB swimmers at his local Masters club and realised that natural swimmers engaged the water, rather than snatched at it; breathed rhythmically, rather than gasped; and streamlined their bodies to slip through the water instead of fighting their way through it.

He studied with the Amateur Swimming Association to learn the theory behind what he was seeing. He became one of the fastest swimmers in his age group – not by being fitter or stronger than the next person, but by using flawless technique. His journey from 'holiday splasher' to fast and efficient open water swimmer prompted him to switch careers, and teach others the mechanics of a fast and efficient front crawl.

Or so it says on his website. I added the bit about him being one of the world's great swimming teachers, because he really is. He's also one of the good guys: friendly, smiley, interested. He once told me some of his clients see him as an avuncular uncle – Avuncular Uncle Ray – and I reckon that's about right (unless you haven't done your drills):

'Swimming really does give you a reset. When I'm swimming, I start by thinking about the technique. Then once I've ticked that box, I can let my mind wander. And when you swim really well, there's a point where I describe it as almost being a passenger in your own body. When you've gone through the process – you've gone through building muscle memory, you've gone through that quite boring, repetitive process – when the stroke clicks you get this constant, relentless, almost effortless flow, which you can do for hours. It's a beautiful place to be in and I love getting that feeling that I'm merely travelling in the vessel which is my swim stroke.'

We're chatting over breakfast before my lesson. I'm scoffing mushrooms with beans on toast while he sips a coffee. There's an iPhone between us recording the obvious passion oozing out of his every pore. Ray adores what he does, adores the sport that's become his living. At one point he mentions the feeling of swimming downhill. Swimming downhill? I almost spit mushrooms all over the table:

'Yep, and I get that on every swim. At some point I'll be feeling it and smiling in the water. This is amazing. Because I don't come from a swimming background, I don't take it for granted. I'm 58 years old and I still get an amazing buzz out of that feeling of swimming well. And that's why I enjoy giving people that. And when they get it, and you'll get it, then I can see that they're like, "Oh my goodness, this is what it's all about." Anyway, when you see someone at the swimming pool who can really swim, you can see that they're getting that. That easy propulsion; that state of grace.'

Right now, I'm about as far away from a state of grace as it's possible to be, thrashing around in the 20-metre pool of a subterranean city gym and attempting the basic extension. All other swimming has, for the time being, been banned. Let's get your stroke right first, says Ray, or you'll be practising your mistakes.

The timing is perfect. It's late November. The water outside is too cold to spend extended periods of time in and my endurance is pretty good anyway from all the running. The winter before my Channel swim is for honing my technique.

Except at the moment it's really not happening.

4

Swimming Bluetits

It's started snowing – big, lustrous, white flakes falling like confetti over a largely deserted South West London – so, obviously, I get in the car and head to the Thames for my second swim of the morning.

Technically this may still be illegal. It's difficult to keep track of the ever-changing Covid restrictions, but even if this 'second exercise of the day' is not within the rules, even if I could technically be arrested, I'm willing to take the risk. Since I've been wild swimming I've been dreaming of a river swim in the snow. The journey is perilous in a tiny car on icy streets, but I refuse to turn back. Today feels like a real waypoint on a journey that began in the same stretch of river less than a year previously.

That first time, there were three of us tentatively entering the Thames about a mile west of Teddington Lock in Kingston. Me, my friend Oli from running club and our mutual friend Marlene. We were (still are) all members of the Serpentine Swim Club. Oli, a former Special Forces soldier and quite resourceful when the mood takes him, had found a place for us to get our open water fix during lockdown when the Serpentine was closed.

We both live in Barnes, where we're at the mercy of tides and sewage leaks, but the river west of Teddington Lock is non-tidal

– and relatively clean – so we could turn up and swim anytime. A pleasant treat when we had literally nothing else to do. We'd meet up – at a time when every opportunity for contact with other human beings was a godsend – strip off in our cars and carefully lower ourselves into the water. In those days passers-by would give you some properly odd looks when they saw you swimming in the river in winter. Actually anytime. We've come a long way very quickly with swimming outdoors.

The usual thing was to get acclimatised to the water and chat for five minutes or so as we swam upstream doing head-up breaststroke. Then Oli and I would transition into a lazy front crawl for about a quarter of an hour while Marlene continued her powerful breaststroke. There's something so wonderful about being in the water and experiencing the ancient River Thames from a duck's perspective, whatever swim stroke you're employing. At some stage we'd turn around and swim back with the flow, all of us reunited for the final few minutes and enthusing about how lucky we were.

Once, the current was so strong we tried to swim upstream and found ourselves going backwards. After that we'd always check the flow before entering and, if necessary, we'd do a one-way swim, starting much further west towards Kingston Bridge. And on the rare occasions the tides and sewage dumps were in our favour, we'd swim in the much bigger tidal Thames in Mortlake, Barnes or Hammersmith.

There the trick is to enter about 15 minutes before high tide and go with the flow until it changes. You've got about five minutes of slack water, after which you come back the way you came, being careful not to overshoot your exit point. If you do, you either face a flat-out upstream sprint to get back to it or a mildly awkward semi-naked walk back to the car from wherever you do manage to exit the Thames.

That's usually the steps opposite Barnes Bridge railway station, the slipway next to the Ship Inn, the corner of

Hammersmith Terrace or the ladders on Lonsdale Road by the Bull's Head pub. The last one is especially satisfying as nobody passing by knows you're about to emerge on to the pavement until your dripping wet, topless torso pops over the wall with towel and clothes dangling behind you inside a yellow dry bag tied around your waist.

One day in Teddington, a woman walking her dog did that 'You lot are mad!' thing, but then asked what it was like in the water. We invited her to join us the following day and she did. All of a sudden, we were four.

The following week, Marlene's Turkish friend Yesim moved into a local block of flats and she came along too. Yesim loudly proclaimed that the cold water made her feel alive like nothing she'd ever experienced. And four became five. Soon we were joined by a Virgin Radio listener who recognised me on the riverbank. And a local teacher, who turned out to be my son's nemesis who kept putting him in detention, a workaholic lawyer who lives nearby, Marlene's friend Ian who had to be surgically removed from his wetsuit. Six, seven, eight, nine...

When we reached double figures, Marlene started a WhatsApp group and called it the Teddington Bluetits after the open water swimming group in Wales which spawned similar groups all over the country. 'Whoever you are, wherever you are from, you can find fun and friendship in our cold water swimming community.' And so it proved in West London. There are now almost 3000 members of Marlene's Bluetits group and she welcomes each new joiner with as much joy and attention as she did when there were fewer than a dozen of us:

'At first people would pass us as we were in the water and say, "What on earth are you doing?" But they could see how much fun we were having and would want to try it too. The next day they were there having bought all the kit, float bags and swimming robes, and caps and goggles. The swim group grew quite quickly.

'Eventually I stopped giving out my number and would just tell people to find us on Facebook. We started to run it through a Facebook group, the Teddington Bluetits, and all they had to do was apply to join. And people loved it and word spread quickly. Friends of friends and people passing. Two and a half years later we have almost 3000 members.

'We're effectively a bench on the river bank in Ham. We're like the Brentford of the swimming world. Brentford, the Premier League football club I support, is famously "just a bus stop in Hounslow". Well, we're a bench on the riverbank. But it is the most beautiful stretch of riverbank. It's non-tidal, it's smaller than the river a few miles away in central London and it's so pretty. It's like country river.

'I set up the WhatsApp group to arrange the swims, but people put a lot of information on there as well about kits and other places to swim. Photographs get uploaded and literally hundreds of messages every day.

'Mostly there are three to four swims a day. When I set up the group, there were three swims a week. I would go to each swim and then, as the group grew, people would just arrange the swims between themselves. The group almost self-manages now. I just suggest events like full moon swims, fireworks swims.'

The Teddington branch of the Bluetits is the friendliest and most welcoming in the world. Everyone says so. Having watched it grow from the start, I can definitely vouch for that. And I can absolutely vouch for the fact that it's all down to Marlene's care, imagination and flair. I once turned up to a night swim to find everyone lying in a circle chanting at the full moon. A woman was walking around with some Tibetan gongs, giving everyone a pre-swim sound bath. It sounds a bit woo-woo, but it was magical. Trust Marlene to think of trying it. She, of course, puts it down to everyone else:

> 'The group is so diverse. We've got such a wealth of interesting people in there. One of them is my friend Dao, who is a sound therapist. She sometimes brings her Tibetan gongs to the riverside and gives us all a sound bath in the dark, under a full moon. It's a really lovely spiritual experience, actually.
>
> 'Full moon swims are a big thing. Every month we make sure we're in the water just before the full moon comes up. Then as we're out, the moon is coming up and we can see it rising above the river on the horizon. We've got bats swooping down on the river to see what we're doing as well and I always bring a trolley.'

The trolley lives in Marlene's sunshine yellow Fiat 500, which she drives around South West London like she's in a Grand Prix. The trolley is almost as much a part of the Bluetits as the river. People make a point of baking for it, not least Marlene, who's so good at making cakes, she was once shortlisted for *The Great British Bake Off*. They call it 'Lakes, drakes, bakes and cakes' and it's a real social event:

> 'We don't just swim and go straight home. We chat, we socialise, we get to know each other. People say that's really important as well. It's as much about the community as it is about the water. We connect with each other. We forge friendships. Especially through lockdown, people just wanted to see other people. Water was a nice environment to do it and friendships have grown. It's been lovely.'

'Lovely' might sound a little lame as a description, especially in an age when everything seems to have to be the 'best thing ever'. But 'lovely' is perfect. Just that feeling of loveliness, being in nature, being eye level in that rippling water, like being in the middle of a Monet painting. And those little swims, every time we did them, they were like a mini adventure. It was, yes, *lovely* to see all the birds on the river, swans flying over us, fish below us, eye level with the little ducklings on the cold, clear water. A couple of times a seal popped up almost next to us. Lovely, lovely, lovely.

Every swim is a tonic, a way of being born again. And each swim is also a question: am I brave enough to take the plunge? You should hear the grumbling on the riverbank before the Bluetits enter the water. 'Oh what are we doing? Oh it's cold. Oh the bank is muddy and slippery. Where am I going to leave my phone? Why are we even doing this?'

But then the moment of immersion and suddenly, 'Oh, this is just lovely.' One of the joys of going in the river is the beautiful simplicity. It's free. It's there. You are in the water. It's very natural. The Thames has been there for centuries, millennia, and you are just a little part of it. You also, as Marlene keeps saying, really do feel very alive:

'Yeah, it does make you feel alive. You breathe into it, the coldness of the water. We all love the absolute freezing coldness of it. We especially love it when it gets to single degrees, because you come out and feel like you can do anything. It's like a supercharge for your body and for your mind as well. You can go in having had a horrible day at work or home, and the water will just melt all those little worries away. Lots of people have said that to me, especially those with super-stressful jobs. They come, have a little swim and they're happy. Everything's at one again.'

I've often wondered, but been a little reluctant to ask, why these swimming groups seem to be predominately made up of women. Often middle-aged women. I carefully put the question first to Marlene, then to Simon Griffiths of *Outdoor Swimmer* magazine, whose house overlooks the Bluetits' riverside bench in Teddington, to Calum Hudson of the Wild Swimming Brothers, who were taught to swim by their granny in a Scottish loch, and finally to world open water swimming champion Keri-Anne Payne. (And, yes, I'm aware that Simon and Calum are men and I asked two males about female participation, but both are swimming experts in a position to give a broad overview).

Marlene:

'I think it's because women are more adventurous. The men in the group will freely admit that as well, although the men who join the group absolutely love it. I suggest coming along to some of my other male friends, but they're like, "Oh goodness! No thanks, not the river." Women are happy to embrace that. Swimming just seems a naturally beautiful thing to do in a natural environment.

'You don't have to be an athlete to do wild swimming. A lot of the group just like to pootle up and down. We don't properly swim. Most of us don't put our head down in the water. We don't front crawl. We breast stroke up and down and chat while taking exercise. It's almost like this naughty, daring thing we're doing. The colder the water gets, the more it feels really exciting. Also, it's non-competitive and that's absolutely key, because anyone can do it. Nobody judges you about how far you go, how fast you go or even how long you spend in the water.

'One couple who come along are Leslie and Michael. Leslie is actually a therapist in a prison and Michael's an author. At one stage Leslie swam pretty much every day, because the river helps melt away the stresses of her job. She bakes for the group. She organises outings to Hampstead Ponds. She absolutely loves the group and that couple, they come together every week. It is been lovely meeting them.

'Meanwhile, there's a high-powered lawyer who works all the hours God sends. She's admitted that she's not very sociable, but when she comes to swim, she'll chat to everyone in the river. She just says it's so peaceful and calming, and it's so opposite of her everyday life. The river, again, is like a therapy for her. It slows her down and also just makes her feel good, just swimming in that water.'

Simon:

'Obviously I've talked to these women. We've interviewed some in the magazine. They write to us at the magazine. I think there's a few things going on. One, a number of these women I've met have never done sport before. They describe themselves as, "Oh, I was never the sporty one at school… I was always the last one to be picked for a team… I was always considered unfit… And then I discovered swimming and discovered I could do it. And I also discovered that actually I can stay in longer than my partner and longer than I ever thought possible for me."

'And they find that it's a very comfortable way to exercise and to move, and to be in nature. And then there's the whole cold water buzz and, although I can't prove this, I suspect that women get more of a buzz out of the cold water swimming than men do. And that's a generalisation. I'm a man, Vassos, and so are you. We both like cold water swimming, love it even, because it's fun. There's a social bit to it as well, but you talk to some women about it and it's like, "That was the most amazing thing ever," which puts it on a different level.'

Calum:

'I think the male ego is perhaps larger and more fragile than the female ego and cold water swimming has a way of stripping the ego bare. You cannot macho or psych yourself through into a cold water swim. You're just going to give yourself hypothermia. So it has a really humbling effect – that you can only swim as far as you're acclimatised. You can only swim as far as you've trained for and that might be increasing by only 30 seconds or a minute every time. The increments are small. It really does humble you. Being cold or getting cold is a different feeling to getting tired or stressed. It has a different effect on your brain, so it really strips the ego. And maybe men are not as comfortable with having their ego stripped away as women.'

Calum's amazing grandmother lived in the wilds of the Highlands of Scotland and was a great inspiration to three active lads, so he and his brothers all have her to thank for their love of wild swimming:

'Bizarrely, our grandma was actually called Grandma Wild, her maiden name was Wild. And she lived up in the highlands of Scotland, incredibly remote, spent her time up and down the hillside or swimming in lochs. From a very young age we had this association of Grandma Wild living out in the middle of nowhere in Scotland and that kind of bled into our childhood as this kind of adventurous outdoor lifestyle.

'It was showing us a soft strength. There was no macho element to how she approached the outdoors. It was more a quiet strength and perseverance. We were very used to seeing grandma swimming in the freezing cold Scottish sea in autumn or winter and that didn't seem strange. She didn't make a fuss about it, she talked about the positives, so when we grew up we didn't think anything of swimming in the local river or the local lake. It felt very normal and natural.

'I'm sure you know what it's like with your kids. If you force them into something too much, it can often send them the other direction. So I think that kind of quiet strength and encouragement was really what showed us that swimming was totally normal, something to be enjoyed, so that helped form our early passion for wild swimming.'

Keri-Anne:

'A lot of women did swim as kids, learned how to swim, and then either work or often family got in the way. We're wired to be very maternal, and rightly or wrongly we take on a lot more than maybe we need to. So a lot of women tend to fall out of any kind of exercise through their thirties and forties when kids are at school. But after the kids leave school we tend to take things on. And swimming has been one of those things, certainly the open water.

'So part one is that it's easy to get back into, it's not like going into the gym which can sometimes be intimidating. But if you see people of all shapes and sizes standing around a lake, there's less worry about you standing around the lake with them. And then there's this community feel. Sometimes you just go down to a lake and notice groups of women standing around chatting together. And it's the combination of that community and being in nature, that's specifically why the open water works. Then the final part is the perimenopause and menopause, which affects middle-aged women. The cold has been a great addition to helping loads of women ease and deal with those symptoms.'

And here's the thing: woman, man, trans, old, middle-aged, young, large, medium, small. Of all the people who've joined us for a swim in the Thames, nobody but nobody has ever regretted it. You *never* regret a swim.

And I definitely didn't regret that day when it was snowing during lockdown and I sprinted to the Thames for my second swim of the day. The journey was hairy, as you'd expect in an underpowered, automatic Fiat 500 on fresh snow. Driving up Richmond Hill was an experience I'm never likely to forget, the little car sliding all over the place as it struggled for grip and traction. Then going down the other side, down Petersham Hill towards Ham, was even worse. I considered abandoning the mission on the grounds of safety and doubtless should have done exactly that, because it was borderline reckless, but the lure of the water proved too strong.

I kerbed the car at the bottom of the hill and briefly thought I'd punctured the tyre. I was hooted long and loud by a van driver who had to take evasive action as I slithered sideways along the middle of the road. I scraped most of the alloys off both passenger side wheels. (My wife Caroline still thinks that was her and I'm literally never going to tell her otherwise.) Eventually, somehow, I got there without injuring anybody. Thank goodness the streets were mostly deserted.

As it turned out, the difficulty and thoughtlessness of the journey served to intensify what followed. I mean, that swim – it sang to the soul. Making fresh prints in two inches of snow with bare feet. Flakes falling from above turning hair temporarily grey. Lying face up in the water, mouth open wide to catch the snow. A white blanket over both river banks. Swans looking camouflaged. The quiet. The cold. The solitude. The water. The joy.

I recently met Craig Foster of *My Octopus Teacher* fame. Over 100 million people watched his Oscar-winning film about diving in the kelp forest off the coast of his native South Africa and meeting a female octopus who cast a spell on him. Craig is one of the gentlest, wisest people you could hope to meet. He told me about something called 'wilderness rapture'.

The previous year he had spent some time with the bow hunters in the Kalahari Desert, who are so connected to their natural environment that they can sense a predator over a mile away, even though they can only see for 100 metres. It's somehow in their very skin. Most of us have lost that deep connection in the tamer world we've created. One such hunter Craig met was walking along, tracking, looking for signs, looking for tracks, no shoes on his feet, thorns on the ground. His life was hard and poor. Survival was the priority every day. And suddenly, this beautiful laughter boiled up inside him and exploded out of his mouth. Craig looked around to see what was funny:

'It would actually happen quite often, but soon I realised it's not something from the outside world. It's simply this primal joy of being in that space and being so connected to the wild. The laughter just comes up. Wilderness rapture. And this is tremendous joy, despite, if you think about it, many of the lives of the people I've worked with, which are very hard and extremely poor, and it's difficult sometimes to survive. Yet there's this extraordinary, innate joy that seems to be connected to being very embedded in the natural world.'

Not wanting to overstate the case, but, yes, there was definitely a bit of that for me in the Thames and the snow. I actually laughed with pleasure, which is as close as I'm ever likely to get – in between Ocado deliveries and dodging London traffic on my Brompton – to wilderness rapture. I bloody love swimming.

5

Swimming Sally

Jersey feels like the right place to be when you're about to start training to swim the Channel. I mean, in all honestly it couldn't really be much further away from the business end, the 21 miles between Dover and Cap Gris Nez. But still, Jersey is very much in the Channel, it's close to France, it has a rich open water heritage, a famous round-island swim, and Sally Minty-Gravett lives there. So when you're entering the sea from the slip at St Catherine's Breakwater, pretending not to be affected by how cold the water is because Sally's watching, you feel like this is perfect.

Fair to say that Sally is a bit of a legend. A string of swimming awards and achievements longer than my weekly shopping list.

In 1965 having only recently turned 18, she successfully swam the Channel. It took her four minutes short of 12 hours – a tremendous time anyway and a staggering time for a teenager. Then in 1985, aged 28, she did it again. And again, aged 35. In fact she completed that third solo Channel crossing days after an 11-hour solo Round Jersey.

She swam the Channel again in her 40s (aged 48 in 2005). And then in 2015, aged 59, she swam from England to France once again. This was a 15-hour continuous swim, and Sally was exhausted when finally her hand felt French sand and she dragged her weary shoulders out of the water on unsteady legs. She enjoyed breathing the clean French sea air for all of four

minutes, ate some peaches and jellies, then dived straight in to
swim back to Dover:

'I did get really worried about the turning around in France.
You're only allowed 10 minutes on French soil. I got over that
when somebody said, "You swim to the start of your swim
and your swim starts when you're in France."

'So I had my jellies and peaches, drank some water, and
also cleaned my teeth, which is a lovely feeling when you've
been in the water for a long time. I re-greased myself because
you're not allowed to be touched or helped. Then I thought,
"Right, I'm swimming back to my husband Charlie," got in
the water, swam back to the boat and carried on to England,
which took another 21 hours.

'I never said at any point, "I've had enough, I want to get
out," because I'd set my mind to swim to France and back to
England. So that's what I did.'

A total of 36 hours and 26 minutes of continuous swimming.
Sally duly became the oldest women to swim to France and
back. The legendary Channel two-way. And she promptly
called it a day. Channel swims spanning five decades, late teens
to late 50s. Sally was rightly awarded an MBE and a place in
the Marathon Swimming Hall of Fame, and had an amazing,
unprecedented string of achievements to take into a hard-
earned retirement.

Only to change her mind in 2022, when she swam to France
AGAIN in her 60s.

Sally is proper Channel royalty and the nicest person you
could hope to meet. And she talks of channel swims as if they're
no more impressive than nipping out for bread:

'Channel swimming wasn't really on my radar growing up,
but I loved being in the sea. My parents were both swimming

teachers and had represented Jersey in swimming and diving, but we didn't have indoor pools until I was 12, when everything changed, because we started swimming through the year. When I was 17, I decided I'd like to do something away from Jersey. I'd already done a couple of six-, seven-mile sea swims with a coach, and I thought I'd go and do Windermere. So in 1974 I went up and did Windermere. Nobody had heard of me. I finished "second lady". And John O'Hara, who was the organiser at the time, said, "You know, lass, if you can do that, you can do Channel."

'So I came home, spoke to my mum and dad, spoke to my coach, and we booked a Channel swim for the following year. It was the centenary year of Channel swimming in 1975, so they were also putting on a Channel swimming relay race to commemorate a hundred years of Channel swimming. We put a Jersey team in. And that's when I met my husband. He was in a pub team, we were the Jersey relay team. We had a fantastic experience.

'Came back to Jersey and two weeks later I go back to Dover, and swim the Channel on the Saturday. I couldn't move for three days afterwards, my arms and shoulders just seized up completely, but I had this inkling that I'd really like to swim from France to England, to say I'd done it both ways, and in 1977 my younger brother swam the Channel and then swam it again.

'I moved back from Canada and trained for a second Channel swim. It was supposed to be France to England, but the wind wasn't favourable, so I did another England–France. My brother and I became the only brother and sister in the world who'd done two England–France Channel swims, but I still had this hankering to do France–England.

'Then in 1991 I was looking after a farmer's kids who were scared of the water. He asked me to teach them to swim and, after I did, he decided to build a big public pool and asked me to run it. That was the stepping stone for me to get another Channel swim under my belt as publicity for opening my swimming school. So on 20 September 1992 I got my France–England swim done, my third Channel swim. We got planning permission to build a pool on the same day.'

I first met Sally on a beach in Jersey where we were presenting the *Breakfast Show* and I was joining a yoga class doing a headstand (don't ask!). Once I was the right way up, she told me she'd be happy to help if I ever decided to swim the Channel and we exchanged numbers. A few months later, she found herself picking me up from the airport (her car seats are dressed up as dry robes[1]) with her adorable dog. Sally and I enjoyed a glorious swim around the bay, then some lunch and a chat, and she kindly agreed to coach me for my Channel attempt the following summer. She also sorted me out with a pilot.

You need an official pilot to swim the Channel – there are around a dozen of them and they're booked up years in advance. An attempt costs about £4000 including the fees for the relevant

---

[1] Dry robes – gosh, where to start. They're obviously a great invention to help keep you warm before and after a swim, especially in winter – basically outdoor changing robes, with thick fleece lining and waterproof shells. You've seen people wearing them everywhere from Windermere to Waitrose. An adult version from the original dryrobe® brand costs £165.

In December 2020, I got wind that Father Christmas would be leaving one under the tree for me and announced the fact gleefully to fellow Serpentine swimmers as we changed outside. I was stunned at their reactions, which ranged from indifferent to disapproving to mildly hostile. That morning was the first time I heard the phrase, 'dry robe w***ers'. Father Christmas had to hastily return my present and buy me a new pair of jeans instead.

Grazia magazine recently described dry robes as 'the must-have, all-season coat', but not all the swimming community agrees. In November 2021 a sign went up on beaches near Dublin saying 'No dry robes allowed' and the slogan 'No dry robes' was spray-painted on a billboard on a beach in Cornwall. At the time of writing, the Dry Robe Owners Club Facebook group has 4500 members. The Dry Robe W***ers group has over 80,000. I still don't own one.

association. Typically, each pilot will have four swimmers per tide. I'd been hoping to be awarded the Serpentine Swim Club guaranteed place. When I wasn't, and feared the attempt would have to be postponed by a year, Sally put me in touch with Mike Oram, who still had slots available (I suspect only because it was Sally who was asking). Sally emailed Mike and Mike emailed straight back. The options were:

11–17 August – Neap tide – no. 3
18–26 August – Spring tide – no. 3
27 August – 1 September – Neap tide – no. 4
10–15 September – Neap tide – no. 3
16–24 September – Spring tide – no. 4
25–30 September – Neap tide – no. 2

Before I could even google the difference between spring and neap tide, and which is easier to swim[2], Sally had picked 10 to 15 September on my behalf.

Suddenly, with a jolt of excited electricity somewhere near my belly button, I realised that this Channel swim was actually happening. I had a date, I had a pilot and I had a coach telling me how little time she had to get me ready. And to stop running. And to find longer pools for the winter miles. And to join swim groups in Dover, Brighton and Dorset. And to start putting on some much-needed brown fat to help with the cold. And to come to her Jersey-based swim camp. And perhaps to have my swim stroke seen to.

---

[2] The spring tide is where the sun and the moon align to create the greatest gravitational pull on the sea. This makes the sea at its most extreme, with the highest high tides and lowest low tides. In contrast, a neap tide is when the sun and moon are at right angles and there is least gravitational pull, meaning the tidal range is at its lowest. I've asked around to the point of becoming annoying and nobody seems to agree which is best for swimming the Channel.

And, basically, I didn't. I'm not much good at being told what to do and quite like being generally haphazard. For instance, I turned up on the start line of my first ultra-marathon without any trainers – I'd forgotten both pairs by the front door – so had to run 62 miles in old gardening shoes (the state of my feet afterwards!). I've never once laid out a 'Flat Stanley' of all the kit I'll need before a big race and therefore forget stuff. I've lost count of how many sea and lake swims I've done without a towel. I'm not a planner, and I like me that way.

I got spooked by all the planning apparently needed for a Channel attempt and reacted in the best way I know how: I buried my head in the sand. Instead of allowing Sally to help and direct all preparations, we agreed to catch up every few months. No swim camp in Jersey, no reduction in running, no longer pools, no outdoor swim groups. I reckoned I'd do it all my way.

Mind you, I did chat to Sally quite a lot. I once asked her about her hardest crossing:

'That was 2005. It was a few years after the French authorities had stopped people swimming from France to England unless you did a two-way, so I booked a two-way. And on the day I was so ill and so sick – we put it down to nerves – that I just did it a one-way.

'Oh, it was horrible. It was only a 13-hour swim. It wasn't a long swim, but I was just really sick for the first six or seven hours. It's probably the closest I'd ever been to being taken out, because every time I became vertical, I thought I was going to pass out. And I thought, "I'm not going too close to the boat in case they hoick me out." I stopped feeding, because it was making me sick again. And after about eight hours, I just went, "I'm not having anything else to eat or drink. I'm just going to finish the swim." And the last four or five hours were without any food or drink.

'When I finished, I was as right as rain. I finished on a sunny afternoon. There was a live broadcast on the local radio of me finishing. Radio Jersey phoned my husband as I was about to land in France and he was talking to them while I was coming out on the beach. And I spoke to them as soon as I got back on board. So that was really exciting. It was fun.'

It's got to be quite a moment when you land in France. When your hand hits sand. I've spent some time trying to visualise that, almost willing it to happen for me. Of course, not everyone will have a husband on a live link-up to their local radio station, but I imagine cheering crowds as you exit the water. And a brass band! A chorus of angels! And, of course, a slap-up French dinner followed by a well-earned night in a posh hotel, but Sally sets me straight:

'No, no, you have to come back. Legally you have to come back. There may be people on the beach out walking their dogs or whatever, and they just carry on walking. If you land in France and there's people walking along the beach, they just watch you land, take a picture if you want a picture and carry on walking. It's funny. They're very nonchalant about it.

'When I finished my two-way and landed in England, that was different. It was probably the hottest day of August. There were dolphins playing on the left, the sun was setting, and I remember vividly looking up at the light and asking the time. It was 5.15 p.m. – exactly 41 years to the minute after my first Channel swim.

'Then I swam into the Leas at Folkestone, because I didn't want any stones or slopes. I needed something where I could stand up easily. Because you have to do it all on your own. You're not allowed to be touched by anyone until you're clear of the water. By then it was about 9 p.m. The sea was like glass. I was giggling incessantly. My vision had started to go, because I was so tired and dehydrated, and I was seeing double, hallucinating a little. I thought everyone had fancy dress on. Really bizarre.

'So I got on to all fours, tried to get up and face-planted into the sand. Got on all fours, face-planted again. And then I turned around and bum shuffled backwards. You're horizontal for such a long time, you have to get your balance before you can stand up. And once I got my balance sorted, then I turned around and stood up and I got the biggest hug. Graham, who was on my boat, he's six foot five, and he just gave me the biggest bear hug. It was just gorgeous.

'Then they carried me on my back, back to the boat, because you're supposed to lie flat straight away, because you have to be very careful with fluid on your lungs when you're horizontal for such a long time.

'My mouth and nose and throat were all so ulcerated I couldn't actually eat or drink anything. I lost the skin on my tongue and I sat in the chair and the only thing Charlie could feed me was ice cream. That took about three weeks to heal. I couldn't have a proper drink of champagne or gin and tonic for at least 10 days, which is a shame, but probably didn't do me any harm!'

Sally coached actor Will Ellis to his successful Channel crossing. He took all her advice and even spent his summer holiday at Sally's house with his family. Sensibly, Will took all her advice and expertise. And Sally was on board his support boat when the wind started howling halfway across the Channel. There was a large WhatsApp group ('Collecting a Pebble from France') of Will's friends and family following his progress with the GPS tracker and updates from Sally. She shared a video of the swell with the caption, 'Will is officially a member of the Force Six Club.'

Experienced swimmers explained to the rest of us just how hard it had become. Ray the swim stroke teacher – who also helped Will – commented that he's seen six-person relays get pulled from seas like that. That, said Ray, was a SWIM! I was thrilled for Will. Nobody deserved a successful Channel swim more than he does. And definitely not someone who didn't even do what Sally told me to.

6

Swimming Downhill II

Ray gets booked up quickly and the first lesson I can arrange is for about a month after I first make contact. He's based in Canary Wharf, in an industrial unit dominated by a small pool rigged with waterproof cameras. Cameras to right of you, cameras to left of you, cameras in front of you... If there's a kink in your stroke, Ray's going to find it.

The pool is around five metres by three and only about a metre deep. There's an endless current coming from a machine at the front, speed adjustable, but only by Ray. Swimming in it is strangely satisfying – a lot like running on a treadmill and quite pleasant for short periods of time. We have a chat, I tell him my news – 'I have a September Channel tide' – and we dive straight in (not literally).

I'd been to visit the legendary Sally Minty-Gravett in Jersey and we had swum together in the harbour. In Jersey she told me she was pleasantly surprised by my technique. Not much to work on, she thought. Almost not even worth going to see Ray. Almost.

Well, thank goodness I did go to see Ray. What Sal couldn't see in St Catherine's Bay, Ray noticed immediately with his cameras. It's a funny thing, the swim stroke. I spent six months thinking of very little else so forgive me if I get a bit technical.

Because here's the thing: it turns out that all of us – you, me, the woman in the floral swim cap sharing your lane at the gym, the bloke splashing around next to you at the leisure centre thinking he looks all serious and 'triathlon' – have been doing swimming all wrong and Ray basically has me going back to primary school to relearn my letters before I'm allowed to do joined up writing:

'You had a typically naïve stroke. You were confident in the water, which is half the battle. With some people, it's half survival, so if you watch them, their stroke is 50% climbing out of the water to breathe and 50% propulsion. You're clearly willing to learn and I was preaching to the converted, because you'd been recommended by some really switched-on people in the channel swimming and open water swimming world. Also, you're a great listener, which probably comes with your job, and you inquire as well, which is great. You test me and make me work for my money, because you ask questions. But yeah, with you I could see it was fairly straightforward. I would teach you the movements with various exercises, and then I knew that you would go away and repeat them.'

Those exercises, though. That first one, basic extension. I struggle to get the hang of it at all. And it's a downward spiral of leaking confidence. If I can't do the very basic thing, what chance have I got with the granddaddy of all swimming challenges? I'm marginally better on my left side and persuade myself that's because I'm blind in my right eye. Perhaps I can't do basic extension, because of my eyesight, I find myself rather idiotically thinking. And then believing.

For the fortnight between my first and second lessons with Ray, I practise basic extension four times for 20 minutes a time. Ray warned me he can always tell when his students don't work sufficiently hard at their drills, but I thought I knew better. Plus

I had the eyesight thing up my sleeve. How many clients are blind in one eye, for goodness sake? 'I've tried my best, but unfortunately I have a physical handicap that prevents me from doing basic extension.'

Avuncular Uncle Ray turns into malevolent Uncle Ray when he sees how little progress I've made. Reminds me that the Channel is not to be trifled with. Reminds me how little time I have to correct my swim stroke. Has absolutely nothing to do with the ridiculous eye excuse:

'If you practise basketball once a week, you're not going to improve. It's as simple as that. You need to practise at least twice a week, three times a week, and that's the bare minimum. Occasionally someone will walk in, they've Googled me in Canary Wharf and they'll walk through the door, but sometimes I still have to eke the motivation out of people.

'There are still a few triathletes who see swimming as an inconvenient way of getting on their bicycle. Once they become good swimmers, and they start to enjoy swimming and they keep improving, then guess what? They find more time to go to the swimming pool, because it's such a lovely thing, going right back to that lovely feeling. So all of a sudden, someone who had no time to do more than one swim a week is doing four swims a week. And then guess what? Quite often a triathlete will start doing 5K or 10K open water swims for the love of swimming.'

I get the wake-up call I needed in that second session. I join a gym with a swimming pool and resolve to do my drills religiously four or five times a week. They're no fun. The expression 'drills are for dentists' exists for a reason, but once you commit, they become oddly rewarding, and occasionally you glimpse where the drills are taking you, to some beautiful far-off horizon, and the monotony becomes worthwhile.

7

Swimming Journey

I've had a little time off work, and done that silly thing and overfilled it. Sleep is such a precious commodity, especially when you start your working day at a time when most normal people are considering one last drink before bed. I need to be careful or I'll arrive back at work more tired than when I left, so frankly the last thing I want to do on my final day off is get up at 4 a.m. to drive to Marlow, board a bus for Henley and swim back to Marlow. Over dinner the night before the proposed swim I decide to pull out, spend a nice relaxed day by the beach in Whitstable, where we have a cottage. I don't need to do this.

So, of course, 4 a.m. comes around and I'm behind the wheel of our electric car, pointing east and fretting about the range. Marlow is 104 miles from Whitstable, a good two hours, and I haven't charged the car overnight, because I didn't think I'd be driving. But it turns out my fear of a Did Not Start almost matches my Did Not Finish phobia. I once gave a talk called 'Do Not Fear a DNF' – to encourage people to get out of their comfort zone – but I had to admit at the outset that I was a bit of a fraud. Because I really DO fear the DNF.

I have just one on my CV and it still hurts. The golfer Doug Sanders was asked, on the 40th anniversary of missing a one-foot putt to win the sport's biggest prize, whether it still rankled with him. 'Oh goodness no,' he replied. 'That was four decades ago. These days I can often go a whole 15 minutes without thinking about it.' It's how I feel about the Dragon's Back Race which, injured, I failed to finish in 2017.

It was the same bit of my brain that, almost on autopilot, set the alarm for 3:50 a.m., despite my earlier promise to myself to catch up on sleep. Now, as I zoom along the M2, other parts of that ludicrous mind of mine are worrying about, in no particular order: whether I have it in me to swim the nine miles between Henley and Marlow, whether to wear a wetsuit, whether last night's raucous supper will adversely affect my swimming, and, of course, whether the car will make it to Marlow and back with a battery which is only 42% charged.

The swim is being organised by the brilliant Henley Swim team. They have another famous event, the Henley Classic, which takes place as dawn breaks over the Henley Royal Regatta course. Dive in at the first hint of sunlight and swim the same 2.1 kilometres which the rowers will compete on later: past landmarks like the Barn Bar, Phyllis Court and Members' Grandstand. As the church and bridge come into sight in the early morning, you end the swim at the Official Regatta Finish. I swam this years ago and if you don't camp on site it involves a ludicrously early start, so at 2 a.m. one Saturday morning, a time which is still Friday night for most, I found myself donning my wetsuit and heading off to Henley.

I'd just driven over Hammersmith Bridge (back when you could) and was about to turn left on to the A4. The traffic lights went orange, I decided to go for it, accelerated, changed my mind, braked hard, changed my mind again, sped up, only to decide at the last second to obey the law and come to a screeching stop. A terrible piece of driving. Unfortunately for me, it happened right in front of a police patrol car, which wasted little time in flashing its blue lights. The uniformed officer slowly walked to my car and I wound down the window.

'Do you know why we've pulled you over, sir?'

'Yes, sorry, that was appalling driving on my part.'

A pause. The officer looks at me quizzically. It's 2 a.m.

'Are you wearing a *wetsuit*?!'

'Erm, yes, but there's a good reason.'

'Do you know what?' said the copper as he started edging away with a look of mild distaste. 'I honestly don't want to know.' And with that, he hurried back to his car and drove away. I often think what he must have thought I was up to wearing rubber at 2 a.m. on a Saturday morning. All of which I recount for no other reason than every opportunity to tell the tale should be taken.

The swim I've signed up to this morning is called the Henley Marathon, the Henley Swim team's blue ribband event and their last of the summer. It takes a lot of effort to ensure a thousand or more people will be safe over a nine-mile stretch of river. The organisers have been hard at it for months. Just as I'm nearing the end of mine, they're about to embark on some much-deserved time off. First though – this.

There are hundreds of people milling around Higginson Park in Marlow, some topless, most wearing wetsuits. We must make for quite a sight at 6 a.m. Everyone is carrying a luminous blow-up bag, because that's the main rule for the morning: tow floats compulsory. It says so front and centre of the website and on every email. They have a clever technical way of forcing you to watch the safety briefing online before you can register. The 'don't forget your tow float' rule must be mentioned half a dozen times during the briefing. I've forgotten my tow float.

This means that in among everything else they've got to do this morning, the organisers have to find and loan me a tow float. They're extremely nice about it, batting away my profuse apologies. And everything runs like clockwork. Swimmers board courtesy coaches, colour-coded with swim caps matching the relevant start wave. I'm in an early wave and in one of the first coaches to set off.

The woman sitting next to me is a veteran of many swim marathons. She exudes confidence and capability. She tells me about her target splits, how she plans to minimise time lost at locks, which landmarks along the route she's particularly looking forward to swimming past and how to minimise mileage by taking the inside line of every bend in the river. She doesn't mean to, but she's making me much more nervous.

We arrive in Henley and meet Tom, who runs Henley Swim. Lovely bloke and a lovely chat. He seems completely at ease on land and in water, despite all the moving parts, across the nine miles that separate Henley and Marlow. Chatting to Tom calms my nerves and I'm feeling pretty chipper as I don cap and goggles, and dive in.

From the moment we start swimming, the morning becomes an absolute delight. There are kayaks to keep us safe and on course. There aren't too many swimmers in the water at the same time so you're not constantly swimming round or over people. And because we're wearing timing chips on bands around our ankles, there's no need for a mass start. We enter the water in ones and twos, so blissfully there's no 'washing machine' effect.

There's not a great flow today, but the current is definitely helping. Worst case scenario, you could lie on your back, using your tow float as a pillow, and let the river gently guide you to Marlow. That's emphatically not what I do. I start swimming hard; hard enough to need to breathe every two strokes rather than my usual three. I find myself wondering, is this better? Should I be breathing like this generally? Is breathing more often better? Would it get more oxygen to the muscles? And come to think of it, what *is* the perfect way to breathe while swimming?

Fortunately, I know a man who knows. Patrick McKeown is the breathing guru's breathing guru. He discovered something called the Buteyko Breathing Technique in his 20s and, after a lifetime of asthma medication and inhalers, found immediate and permanent relief from his symptoms. He travelled to Russia to meet Dr Konstantin Buteyko and promptly set up a company, Oxygen Advantage, dedicated to helping people breathe and feel better, and achieve their potential.

Patrick's big thing is nasal breathing. When I first met him, one of his disciples had just completed the brutal, 60-hour Barkley Marathons in the mountains of Tennessee – which has a Did Not Finish rate of 99% – breathing entirely through his nose. After 10 minutes with Patrick you'll never breathe through your mouth again. Four days after meeting Patrick, I was due to run the London Marathon dressed in a giant minion outfit. It gets very hot and sweaty in there, with no way of wiping your face as you can't get your hands into the costume. Patrick inspired me to run the entire 26.2 miles breathing only through my nose. Which was quite a feat given how much sweat I ended up inadvertently inhaling. However, nose breathing is obviously impossible while swimming. I call Patrick, who explains it to me very clearly:

'Grand. So there's two aspects. One thing about swimming is that swimming naturally imposes a load on your breathing and that's why children with asthma were traditionally told to swim, because it improves your breathing. You don't want your diaphragm getting tired. If the diaphragm gets tired, blood is going to be stolen from the legs to feed the diaphragm. So the first thing to look at would be how do you help to improve diaphragmatic strength, respiratory muscle strength, so that the diaphragm doesn't fatigue?

'The second aspect is about being able to perform physical exercise with less ventilation. So a swimmer, every time they turn in the water to take a breath, they lose propulsion. It's hydrodynamic drag. And if you can train your body to do a distance, maybe instead of taking a breath every three strokes, to take a breath every four or five strokes, that's much more efficient, because you're not losing energy unnecessarily. Also there's less effort. In other words, you're able to make your body perform more physical exercise with less wasted energy.

'So there's the biomechanics, which is the diaphragm – you want a strong diaphragm – but you also want to improve your breathing from the tolerance of carbon dioxide. So you can imagine, when you're on the water, the water is pressing up against you, so there's a load against you from a biomechanical point of view, but also your face is in the water. You feel air hunger because of the buildup of carbon dioxide. Your ability to tolerate more carbon dioxide is advantageous, because you won't have to breathe so much air.

'How you breathe during the day is going to influence how you breathe in the water. So if you do physical training, running, cycling, whatever you do with your mouth closed is going to help you in the water. Now, in the water itself, you can't nose breathe. It's not possible. So you're taking your breath through the mouth and then you're inhaling it across three, four or five strokes. But that can be difficult at the start, because the air hunger is too much and you run out of air. This is where you want to train your body so you can do that without discomfort. Does that make sense?'

Patrick gives me exercises to help. He gets me to take a normal breath in and out through my nose. After the exhale, I'm to hold my nose and jog on the spot for 15 to 20 seconds. Then breathe normally through my nose, feeling my lower ribs move as I do so. And repeat. Slowly my breath-holding times increase as I learn to tolerate what Patrick calls 'air hunger'.

On Patrick's advice I also start a swimming pool breathing regime. Two lengths of a 25-metre pool breathing as normal, every three strokes. Then two lengths breathing every four strokes. Then every five, which is still no problem. Then every six strokes. Then every seven and it's getting quite tricky now.

Every eight is nasty, every nine horrible and, finally, every 10 strokes is proper grim. Then it's back down again. Every nine strokes feels a tiny bit easier than it did on the way up. Every eight is still hard though and then it's sort of fine from seven back to three. Because it turns out that often it's the breathing – or rather the intensity of the breathlessness – that hampers progress during exercise, as Patrick tells me:

'Often an athlete is training all muscles except the main breathing muscle, the diaphragm. And it's also about training the body to cope better with the changes in blood gases. When you breathe in and out through your nose, your nose adds an extra load on to your breathing. Your nose has about 30 functions, including better gas exchange, and better oxygen transfer from the lungs to the blood and also from the blood to the working muscles.

'It's not about the air that's coming into the body. Really, we should be thinking about how much oxygen is getting delivered to the working muscles. You can actually breathe less air into your body and, if your breathing is efficient, you'll get more oxygen delivery to the working muscles. If an athlete has dysfunctional breathing, the oxygen consumption just to support the respiratory system could be 20% of their oxygen consumption.'

None of which do I know as I gaily swim the first few miles out of Henley breathing every two strokes, greedily gulping in all the air I can. After the first lock, I calm down and start enjoying the process, enjoying the tiredness in my shoulders, wallowing in how lucky I am to have arms that ache from exertion. I also start enjoying the scenery.

You don't necessarily think about scenery on a long swim, what with looking down most of the time. But this particular stretch of the Thames is spectacular and the scenery is unmissable, even to a swimmer. I especially enjoy the glimpses of the enormous houses lining the river with their immaculate, sweeping gardens. My favourite has a handsome wooden boat moored by a private pontoon beside a lavish weeping willow tree whose branches kiss the surface of the water. It's a cross between Toad Hall and something out of *The Great Gatsby*.

There's something special about a point-to-point swim. This feels like a proper journey, but elevated. We're going from Henley to Marlow, a well-trodden route. People drive, cycle, go by boat, run it all the time. Very few swim. I immediately resolve to do more 'journey swims'.

The world's oldest swim spans continents. The ancient Greeks (I do love a myth) told of two star-crossed lovers who lived either side of the Hellespont: Hero, a priestess of Aphrodite, lived in a tower by the sea in Europe, while young Leander was the other side of the strait in Asia. Every night Hero would light a torch at the top of her tower to guide Leander as he swam the strait to be with her, before swimming home the following morning. This being Greek mythology, it didn't end well for either of them. One night the weather was wild and windy, and extinguished Hero's torch. Leander struggled in the choppy, dark waves, lost his bearings and drowned. His body was washed ashore and when Hero saw it from the top of her tower, she flung herself to her death in grief.

The poet Lord Byron also loved a myth and he loved a swim, too. He was born with a club foot which gave him a constant limp on land, but he taught himself to become a very strong swimmer. He decided to become the first person since Leander to swim the strait – the five kilometres of water where the Aegean meets the Sea of Marmara in Turkey. In 1810, on his second attempt, he achieved the feat. It took him just over an hour and he was very pleased with himself as he came ashore, pronouncing, 'I plume myself on this achievement more than I could possibly do on any kind of glory, political, poetical or rhetorical.'

Today, the Hellespont is one of the world's most popular recreational swims and thousands flock to Turkey every year to take part. As I swim past another epic riverside mansion on my way to Marlow, I resolve to book to go to Turkey and follow in the footsteps (swim strokes) of Leander and Lord Byron. After all, the most famous rowing club on this stretch of the Thames is called Leander. They have a hippo as their logo and I feel a little like a hippo as I clamber out of the water to walk over the second of three locks.

There's a bit of a queue to get back in and I start chatting with fellow swimmers. Turns out many have already swum the Hellespont. Indeed I'm frequently told that you can't really call yourself an open water swimmer until you've ticked it off (I'm booked for next year). Others have just returned from an equally epic swim between Gozo and Malta. Then there's the Bosphorus Cross-Continental Swim at the heart of Istanbul, which closes one of the world's busiest shipping lanes for a few hours every year. Swimming holidays are becoming a 'big thing'.

My friend Alison is just back from the Caribbean with the biggest of the swim tourism companies, Swim Trek. Alison swam across the 'Narrows', which separate the islands of St Kitts and Nevis Island, the site of many shipwrecks:

'The St Kitts to Nevis race is actually raced by Olympians, so I thought, okay, cool, I'm doing it. I want a challenge. It's like a skiing holiday, when you ski all day and then you come back, and you have a really nice meal and you feel really fulfilled. That's what I love. That's my perfect holiday. I've done something physical, I've seen something beautiful, and I can relax and enjoy the evening.

'We started very early in the morning and I was nervous. I was thinking, "I'm not going to be able to do this." The sea was very, very rough. The waves were so high that you're often, like, "Where the hell was that point we're aiming for again?"

I couldn't see the boat. Sometimes I couldn't see my fellow swimmers. Some people were getting seasick swimming.

'I kept just reaching, reaching... kept stretching and lengthening my stroke, and kept going. And then you stop thinking, you start to blank out and you're just going for it. At some point I was making songs up in my head. I got cramp in both feet. But when I got there, oh my God, such a wonderful feeling. So good. I was like "Yes!" That's what made me so proud. I'm not designed to be a swimmer, but I did it – and I even beat most of my group. There was a lovely atmosphere among everyone on the swim holiday and it was wonderful to have a journey at the end of it.'

Swim holidays have become big business. Swim Trek alone offers hundreds of different holidays in dozens of countries all over the world, everything from leisurely splashing about in Mexico to ultra-distance training camps in Croatia. Alison was soon spending a week in Oman swimming off a dhow amid dramatic fjords and the cliffs of the Musandam Peninsula.

'Absolutely stunning. Grey-brown mountains plunging into crystal clear, blue water. So beautiful, you just need to be in the water. Some days really rough, some calm as anything. One day we had dolphins.'

And I was booked on a Channel training camp in Minorca with a group called the King's Swimmers... Day four: six-hour sea swim. Day five: 10-hour sea swim. Day six: six-hour sea swim. I was gutted when I had to pull out at the last minute because of a bereavement.

Turn the epic swim dial even further towards 'extreme' and that's where you'll find Dr Julie Bradshaw. She started young, back when she used to go on caravan holidays with her parents in the Lake District. She'd just turned 12 and saw a sign advertising a 'Cross the Width of Windermere' swim: a mile and a quarter, which she swam head-up breaststroke. The following year, when she was 13, she did it front crawl and her passion just grew from there, because, she says, 'Well, obviously, the longer the swim, the better. The colder the water, the better.'

She first swam the Channel at 15. Then she did it again using only butterfly stroke and broke the previous world record by over nine hours. Her other swims include a 29-mile butterfly swim around Manhattan and a 42-mile four-way Windermere in just over 21 hours. She was the first woman to achieve this feat.

She was secretary of the Channel Swimming Association for over a decade, she's a teacher, a sports coach, a councillor and the new Mayor of Charnwood in Leicestershire. She might just be the busiest person in Britain and absolutely impossible to pin down for an interview. Fortunately for me, her wi-fi broke one morning and she had to wait at home for an engineer to come and fix it. I saw my moment and squeezed into her diary. She told me:

'I love swimming. It's like the go-to if there's things going on, stress or anything, just go swimming. Really, really good for mental health. I've got a friend who's medically trained and she talks about all the benefits. It is just amazing, really. There's just something about being in water. A couple of years ago, I contracted costochondritis, which is inflammation where your ribs join the bone in the middle of your chest. I couldn't walk very far and couldn't actually swim, even lying on my front. But I had to get in the water, just even floating in the water. There's something about being in that medium of water, if that makes sense.

'With running, obviously there's you and the environment outside. Whereas with swimming, there's the water all around. You've got your hat on. I wear earplugs. I think most swimmers wear earplugs and it's the melodic tones in the water. And then you've got the waves if you're outdoor swimming. And then depending on what sort of swims you do, for example, like at Windermere, you've got the scenery. With the Channel, it's a slightly different ballgame, because all you get to see for quite a long time is the boat. But on a clear day you can see from England to France, although when you're at water level, it's quite difficult to see ahead.'

Julie and I enjoy a lovely chat about swimming for about 25 minutes while she's stuck at home with no wi-fi. Unfortunately my phone fails to record a large section of it. I notice the glitch just before we wrap up the conversation and hastily press 'record' again just in time to ask her about that wonderful feeling of a point-to-point swim. And also, please could she impart some inspiration for us mere mortals:

'If you believe you can do it, then you can. It's about taking action and most of all believing in yourself, believing that you can do it. And for me it's also about the swimming journeys. I started out when I was young. I'm originally from up north, up in Blackpool, and they used to swim between the piers. Just before Covid, I brought the swim back. The Blackpool Pier to Pier Swim. Two miles between the North and South Pier, taking in the sights of the Golden Mile and Blackpool Tower. Dolphins are sometimes seen in the water. It's a famous, iconic journey and people absolutely love it. But in answer to your inspiration question, the key is to believe in yourself.'

Which brings me neatly back to Marlow. I'm loving every second of this Henley Marathon and honestly can't remember what I was nervous about. I begin to believe in myself. Perhaps I'm not such a duff swimmer after all.

The swim is punctuated by three locks along the nine-mile route and we all exit the water to walk around them. Some run. Others take a leisurely pitstop. The organisers provide everything, from bananas to crisps, energy drinks to chocolate bars. It's seriously tempting to hang around eating and chatting. Everyone seems to have swimming stories up their wetsuit sleeves and a burning desire to tell them.

However, the lure of returning to the water proves too strong. I end up spending only slightly longer at every lock than the Strava brigade, who haul themselves out of the water, sprint around the lock while supping on an energy gel and dive back in barely breaking stride. I'm not after a time, but I'm having a brilliant time. All too soon, a woman on a kayak is telling me I've overshot the finish and now need to swim back upstream to exit the water in Higginson Park. I sort of did it on purpose. I honestly didn't want the journey to end.

Out of the water, medal, photo for the local paper (whoop!), stick around to cheer others home, lose car key, find car key under a gazebo (phew!) and get back on the motorway to Whitstable. It's the opening weekend of the new Premier League season and normally the radio commentary would carry me happily all the way home, but for some reason I can't concentrate on football. I'm reliving the swim and plotting new aquatic adventures, a huge smile on my face.

I make a mental note to talk to my friend Sean Conway. The king of the adventure journey, be it swimming, cycling, running or all three, Sean has cycled around the world and completed 105 Ironman triathlons in 105 days. He once swam – *swam* – the length of Britain, from Land's End to John O'Groats. I've got to leave the final word to Sean:

'We had this map of Britain that we printed out. It was an A1 map, pinned to the door of the boat on the inside. We'd mark off every day and after a month of swimming, I was like, "Wow! I've still got a long way to go." Other than just being cold, I remember having this overwhelming feeling that this is going to take a long time. Even after the first week,

I already knew it was going to take me nearly double what I thought it would.

'I didn't know whether the crew would stay with me. I'd promised them this two-and-a-half month adventure on a boat up the British Isles. It sounds very romantic, but then within a few weeks it looked like it might be an October finish and even that I missed.

'So every day I was not only doing the swimming, always with the current, but I had to somehow make it fun for the crew, which sometimes I did well and then sometimes I was just too exhausted. The crew fed off my energy and if I was grumpy, that'd get them grumpy. And if I was grumpy too much, they'd be like, "Sod this. This is crap. I'm out."

'It was swimming and just ticking off the days every day. Every now and then I'd do a bigger day, say 20 miles, because there was good tide. Those are the days when the line on the map was slightly longer. I'd do a monster day and I'd be like, "Wow! This is huge," and then two days later I'd just have choppy water and I'd be back down potentially to single figures on a bad day.

'The exciting bit was trying to make it an adventure. Yes, it was a physically difficult challenge, but I still wanted to somehow have a fun journey from A to B and see Britain from the coastline, which not many people get to do.

'And I remember, even at the time, feeling privileged to have that view of the land. Very few people get to look at Britain from a mile offshore. You see the cliffs and the birds and... And because the waves were coming from my left, I'd only breathe to the right, which also allowed me to look at the shore, up the entire coastline of Britain. Wonderful!'

8

Swimming Marathon

The guy doing the race briefing keeps cracking weak jokes and it's really helping calm my nerves.

Weak Joke #1: *Has anyone swum this event before?* (A few neoprene-covered arms are raised proudly into the cloudless lakeside sky.) *Well what on earth possessed you to come back and do it again?!*

This is my first 'swim marathon' and the trouble is I'm not feeling 100%. I entered on a whim on Thursday, three days ago, and almost immediately the glands in my neck swelled up – were they rebelling? – and my throat started hurting. I've taken it easy for two days and the lurgy is on its way out, but it's definitely still lurking. What if I swim myself back into the sick bay?

And you know, maybe this whole swimming thing simply isn't meant to be. Three weeks ago I was supposed to be in the Lake District swimming the length of Windermere. I paid for race entry, overnight hotel and return trains. Only for the railways to go on strike and my wife, very unfortunately, to break her elbow.

Now with time running out in the swimming season (it'll be too cold for long swims soon) I've entered a shorter race and promptly fallen sick. Is the universe trying to tell me something?

Weak Joke #2: If you see two beady eyes above the surface of the water, that'll be the famous Dorney crocodile. Swim like hell the other way!

I'm not massively scared of the distance – 10k. More, I'm interested to know how long it'll take me to swim it. I've run 10k in 40 minutes and rowed it in 38. I literally have no idea how long it will take to swim.

I asked in the changing tent earlier and nobody seemed willing to give a definitive answer. The bearded guy changing nearby tutted, the two brothers earnestly downing gels laughed, and the woman at registration said simply 'it depends'. The best answer comes from the bloke I rather awkwardly followed into the bushes for a pre-race pee. He tells me while struggling to do his wetsuit back up that a 10-kilometre swim takes 'about as long as it takes to run a road marathon.' So, anything from three to five hours? 'Exactly.'

Blimey. Five hours? I find myself hoping once again that I don't come last – just like before the Solent swim. I'm new to all this. My confidence is therefore pretty low. The course is two laps of Eton Dorney lake. It was the venue for the rowing events at the 2012 London Olympics so we're not short of inspiration. The lake is just over 2 kilometres long. You swim up to the top corner hugging the left shore, then diagonally part-way down and back up in an M shape, then all the way along the opposite shore. That's halfway.

Weak Joke #3: When you reach this pontoon again, many of you will start identifying as 5k swimmers. That's absolutely fine. Just exit the water and go and have a cup of tea. Nobody will think any less of you. The rest of you – lunatics! – go and do the same again.

He makes a good point. I haven't told anyone I'm here and I could simply call it at halfway if I'm not feeling well. Nobody needs to know. But even as I'm thinking that, I know it's not going to happen. I'm not going to accept the race director's kind offer of transitioning into a 5k swimmer. My only DNF in any race came three days into a five-day ultramarathon in Wales, the world's hardest mountain race, and they literally had to escort me off the mountainside with an ankle the size and shape of a small car.

The thing with me is, I don't give up. It's the only proper positive I've got going for me. But it's massive, a lesson I learnt 20-odd miles into my first running marathon in Barcelona. I was spent. I hadn't done the proper training. My mind was looking for excuses and my legs were running through treacle. All of a sudden the route took us past the open doorway of the hotel I was staying in. The temptation to stop running the race – and start running a bath – was overwhelming.

Somehow I resisted and in that moment mastered the one rule that's driven me to every finish line I've ever aimed for (except that one in Wales). Just keep going – to the next mile marker, street corner, lamp post. Then go again. If you take 'give up' off the menu, all that's left is 'carry on'. I'm hoping – and trusting – that my mantra works just as well in the water as it does on land. Just keep going. And please don't let me be last.

Weak Joke #4: *Those of you towards the rear of the field will encounter swimmers doing the shorter distances. Please be courteous. Don't swim over each other. And move aside if you need to. And remember, everyone else thinks you're mad! Good luck!*

Be courteous. I mean, obviously I'll be courteous and won't swim over anyone. Is that even a thing in a race this long? Yes, I know it's common in sprint triathlons, but a swim marathon? Surely there's more of a sense of 'all in this together'.

I think back to my triathlon days (all four of them). The so-called washing machine at the start of the swim. A sea of garish rubber caps. Arms and legs all over you. Hands using your head as a flotation device. A blur of swimming and controlled drowning. Trying to stay calm, but panicking ever so slightly. Then panicking quite a lot and considering quitting before you've even properly got going. All the fun of the fair. Surely it's not going to be like that.

Okay everyone, if you move forwards and get into the water please, we'll set you off in the next minute or so.

I could have done with another weak joke. I'm beginning to get proper nervous. I look around hoping for an encouraging smile. It's difficult to read expressions under swim caps and goggles, though. Everyone looks very focused.

On your marks... Set... The blast of an air horn gets us underway.

I've positioned myself to the far left of the group, about midway through the field, hoping to stay out of trouble and have a calm start to what will be my longest ever swim. Not a chance. I'm too near the front and it turns out swimming is no different to running – people always start too quickly. I'm swum over multiple times, dunked twice. I fight the rising panic by breathing with every stroke. Good to get the oxygen on board while your stomach's churning and your brain's going 'swimming really isn't for you'. It helps.

Slowly, too slowly, the field spreads out and my breathing returns to normal – every three strokes. There's nothing further to fret about and I settle into a pleasant rhythm. Stroke-stroke-breathe right. Stroke-stroke-breathe left. Just me and the water and my thoughts. In a running race there are things to look at, landmarks, spectators, scenery. Occasionally you'll share a quip, a drink, an encouraging glance with your fellow runners. None of that here. Just the unrelenting darkness of the murky waters and the unchanging lakeside reeds. When you do see a fellow swimmer, hidden behind swim cap and goggles and gulping in air, it's impossible to read their expression. So your only option is introspection. And trying to stop swimming off in the wrong direction, which is proving tricky.

The course is marked by huge inflatable buoys every few hundred metres. It should be easy enough to simply aim for those, but not for a novice like me. I keep veering off towards the centre of the lake, or the edge, and inwardly curse myself for the extra metres I've had to cover getting back on track.

Eventually I get used to 'spotting' where I'm going. I breathe forwards every five or 10 breaths and take a sneaky look at where I'm aiming. It's not perfect, but does mean I can relax back into that agreeable rhythm. Stroke-stroke-breathe. Stroke-stroke-breathe. I'm simply present. In my body and out of my mind. Occasionally a worry will drop into my brain. How far is there still to go? Am I swimming fast enough? Am I going to be ill afterwards?

And so I think back to the conversation I had with one of the great 10k swimmers of all time, Keri-Anne Payne. Our paths have crossed several times since she retired from marathon swimming as a two-time world champion and Olympic medallist. She once came to shadow me at the BBC and we presented the sports news together. We've been patrons of the same charity. And we'd recently shared a stage at an adventure festival where we were both invited to give our thoughts on open water swimming. I felt a bit of a fraud in her presence. Actually a LOT of a fraud. Still turned up mind.

The previous afternoon, as I struggled with a sore throat and butterflies, I'd phoned Keri-Anne for some inspiration ahead of my debut in the distance she made her own. What did she like about swimming 10 kilometres in open water?

'For me it's like an amazing freedom and I love that. I love being out in water that's not so regulated. Swimming pools are so standardised, chlorinated. There's lifeguards. But there's something wonderful about being in any body of water that's uncontrollable, unpredictable. You have to have your wits about you, which is a nice way of being, I think. You've got to think about the wave coming and the chop, and then there's some weeds or there's animals or there's waves. All that kind of stuff, I love it! I'm at my happiest when I'm in the sea. Any sort of sea scenario, I'm delighted with that. Lakes and rivers, too.

'Waves are my absolute favourite. I remember doing a photo shoot for Dry Robes in St Agnes in Cornwall and the waves were bumping. I hadn't been in the sea for ages and I was going through a really tough time in my relationship at the time. And it was the first time I'd been out to the sea for ages and I felt pure joy. I felt like a kid just going in the waves, and then jumping and trying to body surf back in. And it was a real reset mentally for me as well. And I think the open water, especially the sea, really is a consistent place where you know you'll get that.

'Because people can contact us constantly and we're constantly needed. As a mum or a dad or a friend or sister, a brother, a daughter, it never stops. But when you go into the sea, you have to have this level of respect for something that you can do nothing about. I can't change the sea. I can only change whether I go in it or not.

'And also because we're at the top of the food chain and it's just fun I think. It's probably one of the only times in those scenarios where you do something that scares you a little bit. You can know there's no sharks around Cornwall, but there's still that kind of moment of, "Could there be something there?" We are at the will of the ocean and the waves.'

Remembering Keri-Anne's words fortifies my mind and strengthens my resolve as I decide not to swim the extra 20 metres to the far end of the lake, where the organisers have set up a floating aid station offering chocolate, sweets, drinks, crisps. Like any endurance event, aid stations look like the food table for a toddler's birthday party. I swim the M shape around the buoys at the far end and begin heading along the opposite bank back towards the start.

Which is when I start needing to wee. Hardly a big deal. This happens loads on long runs and usually the feeling disappears after a few minutes. Today it only gets worse. I try to shake it out of my mind. What a ridiculous, trivial thing to be troubling me. But soon it becomes all-consuming and my full bladder is all I can think about. Am I allowed to wee in the lake, I wonder? I file the thought under 'who cares' as the need quickly becomes urgent. I decide to wee inside my wetsuit while continuing to swim (saves time, makes it less obvious what you're doing). Remember to wash the wetsuit after, obvs. I try, but it's tough, relaxing the required muscles while working others. I try, I try, I try my best and nothing comes.

So I swim to the side of the lake, stand among the reeds with the water still up to my chest, and try again. It's like standing at the urinal next to the school bully. I'm desperate to empty my bladder, but my bladder's simply not playing ball. I consider climbing out of the lake and finding some bushes. What are the rules about exiting the water during a swimming race? Does doing so disqualify you? I can think of a few reasons why it would. Mainly, because you could re-enter the water further along the lake. And during a Channel crossing you're disqualified if you so much as brush against your support boat.

I abandon my toilet stop and revert to plan A. Ignore the feeling downstairs. The urge to wee will surely go away. How can something so trivial have become such a huge issue? I tend to have little sympathy for people who allow blisters to derail an ultra run they've trained hard for. Blisters are just part of the endeavour. Is needing a wee the swimming equivalent? Am I really going to let this beat me? All that talk about never giving up and I'm being sent potty by, well, the need for the potty.

There are distance markers on this side of the lake, every 250 metres. I'm around halfway back up the lake, just past 750, about 1250 to go until halfway and in serious distress. The fact it's such a seemingly trivial problem only adds to my misery. Please wee, I hear myself begging of my bladder.

I let out a scream underwater. It starts from my toes and by the time it leaves my mouth it's like a volcanic eruption. I imagine the sound travels out of the lake into Maidenhead and beyond. Across the rest of Buckinghamshire, out towards the North Sea, over Scandinavia and into Russia. Vladimir Putin is turning to his nearest lackey and asking what the bloody hell was that? Farmers on the Siberian steppes are crying. Astronauts on board the International Space Station think they're under attack.

By the edge of the lake, I stop again to try to wee in the wetsuit. The scream seems to have done the trick. Unlocked something. I finally begin to pee. The relief, the warmth spreading around my middle, is like nothing I've ever experienced. Not wanting to get too graphic, but the flow seems to go on for eternity. Loads of people swim past oblivious (I hope). How can I have needed that so badly having barely drunk all day?[1] I swim on with a huge grin on my face. I reach the exit pontoon and go past without so much as a thought of transitioning to a 5k swimmer. I've got this. And I'm finally enjoying myself immensely.

---

[1] I was curious to find out what was going on with my body – why I wanted to pee when I was in the water – and I discovered some answers in an article written by open water swimmer Elaine K Howley on the US Masters Swimming website. Elaine reassured me that it wasn't just my imagination – other people had a strong urge to pee when they were swimming, too, particularly in open water.

It's called immersion diuresis and she explained that there are two main factors at play. Being fully immersed in water creates 'hydrostatic pressure' on your body, which increases your blood pressure and signals to your kidneys to filter more and more fluid – hence you need to pee.

When the water you're immersed in is cold, blood rushes to your core to keep your vital organs warm. However, that increase of fluid in your core also indicates to your kidneys that your body's fluid balance is out of kilter, so they go into overdrive and start filtering even more fluid – hence you need to pee even more. So now I knew.

Back up the other side in among the swimmers doing different distances (2.5k, 3.8k, 5k), overtaking and being overtaken, and trying to send out positive vibes to all. The need to wee begins to grow again in my bladder and when it becomes too much, I successfully stop, stand in the shallows and do the business. Making a mental note to learn to 'go' on the go.

Two kilometres later, I reach the floating aid station at the far end of the lake and decide once again not to stop. Many seasoned swimmers have deposited gels and nutrition bottles along the shores – and indeed stored whatever they need on the pier so the volunteers can hand it to them as they swim up. I reckon I know better. The thought actually crosses my immensely stupid brain that as an experienced endurance runner, I can easily cope with three hours' exercise without taking on board extra calories. Not long to go now, I reason. What's the worst that can happen?

The answer is an underwater wall. During a running marathon, this is what they call it when you slow down dramatically once your glycogen stores – your muscles' batteries – run out and you start to rely on fat as a fuel source. The good news is, however skinny you are, you have enough fat to run on for days. And the bad news? It's horrible.

Hitting the wall can also mean a general feeling of cramp, exhaustion, overwhelm. Energy and adrenaline will be running low. Especially when you're not used to it. Keeping those glycogen stores topped up through the race will help, as my fellow swimmers had worked out.

For me, though, having blithely refused all offers of food, I can only draw from the well of my own willpower and guts it out. Which is exactly what I do. The final two kilometres are ugly. Those markers every 250 metres sag, and decide to get further and further from each other until they're miles apart. I'm being overtaken much more frequently now. I'm becoming grumpy. Underwater self-pity, self-doubt, despair, inadequacy. And I've nobody but myself to blame.

Some Shakespeare I learned at school pops into my mind: 'I all alone beweep my outcast state/And trouble deaf heaven with my bootless cries/And look upon myself and curse my fate.' The lovesick subject of Sonnet 29 has his girlfriend to console him and I've got the finishing line. After three hours and 20 minutes, I reach it.

Finally, shoulders sore and needing yet another wee, I emerge exhausted and famished from the water. I towel myself dry, demolish the cake and tea on offer in the tent, and reflect rather fondly on the race. In fact, the ludicrous bladder worries, and the self-inflicted suffering during the final 45 minutes, only enhanced the overall experience. What's the point of doing an endurance event if it's easy. I refuse to berate myself for being haphazard about preparation or a race plan. It's just who I am and, honestly, I do enjoy a period of struggle. Retrospectively. 'For thy sweet love remember'd such wealth brings/That then I scorn to change my state with kings.'

There's a race called the Sri Chinmoy Self-Transcendence 3100 Mile Race. It's held annually around the same nondescript block in the New York borough of Queens and consists of 5649 identical laps – alongside a freeway, around a high school and past a toddlers' playground, with everyday life going on around you. The runners have 52 days to complete the distance, running from 6 a.m. to midnight, and need to average 60 miles every day. The prize is typically a T-shirt or a DVD. The aim is to move beyond ego and, as the name implies, transcend.

I know it sounds weird – and perhaps a bit woo-woo – but in some small way, a long, hard swim brings a similar glimpse of enlightenment. The struggle seems to strip away the layers and connect you with some primal force within. You emerge from the water a tiny bit reborn. And then you scoff cake. Perfect.

9

Swimming Downhill III

We head to Mauritius over Christmas. Holiday of a lifetime. Gorgeous hotel by the sea. Eye-watering price. A fitting celebration of 25 magical years of marriage. We spend Christmas Day swimming with dolphins, Boxing Day building sandcastles. The water is a brilliant azure blue, the beaches simply perfect. And I spend a whole heap of the holiday doing my swim drills.

Up at dawn and creep out of the hotel room clutching flip flops and goggles. Make straight for the sea, a moment to appreciate the sheer wonder of the Indian Ocean. Marvel at how warm the water is, then straight into Ray's homework. He uses Dropbox as his tool of choice. While you're being filmed in his tank in Canary Wharf, he saves your swims, and gives you feedback and pointers via a voiceover track. And most importantly, there's always a homework file to get your teeth into between lessons.

By now I'm in the groove with all the drills. I don't dare skimp on my homework again, not after the admonishment Ray dished out last time. My lessons are on a Thursday morning, every other week, and the following day I'll sit down with a cup of tea in the reception area of my gym and go through whatever's waiting for me on Dropbox. It's like an electronic warm-up.

Often I'll struggle to find the right file and once, somehow, sent Ray my VAT return as I searched for it. Not the first time he's been sent personal files accidentally by clients. A celebrity from *The Only Way is Essex* would routinely upload embargoed publicity pictures. And one city banker sent Ray compromising photos of himself and someone who turned out to be not his wife.

Anyway, my homework file for the festive fortnight involves more basic extension. Lying sideways in the water with one arm stretched in front of you, kicking your feet and trying to feel like you're not drowning when you turn your head to breathe. But there's an extra element this time. Every few seconds bend at the elbow so your arm makes a right angle and your forearm is vertical in the water in front of your face. This is the 'catch'. This is crucial.

If you swim with a straight arm, it takes until that arm is parallel to your chest before it gives you any forwards momentum. Until then, you're doing a lot of work to push water downwards. And you're predominantly using your shoulder muscles to do it and your shoulders are smaller muscles which tire quickly. Better to use your lats.

The latissimi dorsi are the biggest muscles in your back, two triangular slabs found just below the shoulder blades, and extending along the spine down to the pelvis and along the width of the back. You use them if you do a pull-up. They're much stronger than your shoulders, so swimming using your lats just feels much easier. Also, if you're 'catching' the water early, thanks to your 'early vertical forearm', you're extending the stroke – basically propelling yourself further forwards for longer with far less effort.

The catch is what most swimmers go to Ray to learn. Here's his voice track as he filmed my first ever swim. Note the 'praise sandwich':

'You have a lovely minimal turn of the head when you breathe. You'll see swimmers at your gym looking up at the ceiling. From above, I can see excellent length at the back of the stroke, making the most of each stroke. We'll work on your catch. I'm not going to critique your arm recovery or your hand entry. That will change when we change what's going on beneath the water. That's very normal. But that zip on your shorts moving from side to side shows how you've got rotation all the way down through the hips. I like that very much.'

The catch is the holy grail. These early drills are designed to make the elbow bend feel normal and to promote muscle memory. After a lifetime of swimming with my shoulders I've got to get used to bending the arm early and using the lats to propel me forwards.

I commit massively to the drills. For 40 minutes every morning I'm in the shallow waters off the north-west coast of Mauritius kicking the legs, bending the arm, trying to escape the panicky feeling of not enough oxygen. Every third arm bend, you complete the stroke so you're lying on the other side trying not to feel like you're drowning. Also, obviously, trying not to think about sharks. Everybody knows sharks are most active at dawn and dusk, and there are definitely sharks in the Indian Ocean. I fret about it a little every morning, but don't ever see one.

Straight after the morning drills session, I swim for at least an hour. I try to keep concentrating on the catch, try not to revert to shoulder swimming. Occasionally my mind will wander and I'll start enjoying the swim. Fatal. It means I've lost focus and forgotten about the catch. Never forget the catch!

After almost two hours in the sea I feel like I've earned the enormous hotel buffet breakfast. And then later I'll find the time to train again, same as before, drills and a swim. Every day. Even on a swanky holiday. Practise, practise, practise. Drills, drills, drills. In the dying light of the early evening, I do my drills in the large hotel pool with families cavorting all around and bats flying overhead. How wonderful, I keep thinking. This time next week I'll be back in the small subterranean pool in central London. And back under the unforgiving gaze of Ray's cameras. At least this time I'll have done the work and I'm beginning to get it right. Although, as it turns out, I'm not getting it right at all.

10

Swimming Pool

How many people can say they're transcending at their local David Lloyd? I want to get a long swim in and don't have time to drive to the sea or a lake, so I take advice from an *Eastenders* actor, drive to Raynes Park, and get stuck in.

The actor is Will Ellis, who plays Theo Hawthorne in the soap, and he's a proper swimmer. When we first chat, introduced by the irrepressible Sally Minty-Gravett, who's been helping us both with our swimming training, he's just back from swimming around her native Jersey, a cool 44 miles. He only just failed to break the record, and only because of bad luck with tides and shipping. He hosts the popular *An Open Water Swimmer's Podcast* and generally loves everything to do with this wonderful, madcap sport.

During that first chat, Will mentioned something brutal he uses for training called 'a hundred hundreds'. You do one hundred 100-metre swims, going on timed intervals, every 90 seconds in his case. I give myself two minutes and even then don't manage much rest between sets. That comes to three hours and 20 minutes exactly for what will eventually be 10 kilometres.

The David Lloyd at Raynes Park, next door to the Wimbledon's All England Tennis Club where its founder once reached the semi-finals, is epic. The biggest and best gym and spa you'll ever see, and two swimming pools, a 25-metre indoor and a 20-metre outdoor. Those five metres make a hell of a difference when you're swimming a long way, but I opt for the outdoor pool, because it's less busy and, frankly, it's just nicer to be in the open air, even on a drizzly spring morning like this.

This will be my first long swim of the year, after I've spent the winter honing my new stroke. Teacher Ray has taken a month off and sent me the usual homework file via Dropbox. The drills are still there, some kicking and basic extension to start, half an hour of the advance single arm drill with a flat paddle and then, in Ray's words 'a long swim'. When he says long, he probably doesn't mean over three hours, but since he didn't explicitly say not to, I decide I'm fine to go ahead. With my potential Channel swim less than five months away I'm becoming increasingly anxious about it and reckon a successful long swim will calm the nerves.

So that Saturday morning I arrive at around 7.30 a.m., change speedily and head outside. There are two lanes, fast and slow, encompassing about half the surface of the pool, and the rest is clear water. There's one person using the slow lane but – and this is a good tip – I reckon I'll be least disturbed if I swim in the open, lane-free section of the pool and hog the edge of the lane marker. I'm proved emphatically right. Both official lanes soon have two or three swimmers in them, either splitting the lane or going around clockwise at the speed of the slowest swimmer. Meanwhile, my section does fill up, but I'm left to my own devices as I go up and down, up and down, next to the floating blue and white (with red ends) divider.

But. Oh. My. Goodness. The sheer, complete and utter, mind-numbing, total, all-encompassing, all-consuming BOREDOM!!!

Quite recently, I almost lost my rag with someone who told me they didn't want to run a marathon 'because they'd be too bored.' It was the most pathetic excuse I thought I'd ever heard. They'd be too bored? *Too boring*, more like. Well, I take it all back. Have you ever tried swimming 10k in a 20-metre pool? It's excruciating. Stroke by stroke, your very soul is progressively anaesthetised.

Set your watch timer for two minutes and set off swimming. Five lengths. Try not to push too hard off the edge of the pool each time as that feels like cheating. Finish at the opposite end from where you started. Look at your watch, realise you've gone far too fast, wait almost 30 seconds for the stopwatch to reach 2 minutes and set off again. Five more lengths. Better this time, nice and easy, around 1:45. Give yourself 15 seconds of rest then you're back underway.

Try to remember the correct stroke, the catch, the rotation, the leg kick, the noodle arms, the elbow dink. Too fast again. Settle down – 300 metres is only 3% of your total swim. Try not to think about that fact too much as you catch your breath and wait for the second hand to tick up to six minutes. Then go again.

Why are you already feeling tired? Why is your shoulder aching? Finish after barely a minute. Realise you're two lengths short and go again. Only 10 seconds to rest this time. Seems like you've already been in the pool for ages, yet you're only one 25th of the way. If this was a road marathon you'd be passing the one-mile marker. Keep going, this has got to get better. Can't get any worse. Gets worse.

The fifth 100-metre set hurts your shoulders and also leaves you gasping for air like you're going too quickly – but you finish almost exactly at the two-minute mark. After three miserable seconds contemplating your life choices, you go again.

Maybe you don't need to finish this? After all, it's not part of the training plan. Do a few more reps, maybe even swim up to a total of two kilometres and call it a day. You'd then have time to take your nine-year-old daughter to netball. Be a better dad. Another set done, 10 seconds to rest, off again.

Yes that's exactly what you'll do. Get to 20 sets and call it a day. Probably for the best as you don't want to be practising any mistakes. You should only do a long swim when Ray explicitly suggests it. That's seven down now. Get going on number eight. Why is that shoulder of yours still hurting? Have you got an injury? Picked up in the gym perhaps, when you were playing around on the monkey bars pretending you were an actual monkey. That would be typical, wouldn't it? Monkeying around and ruining your dreams and aspirations in the process. How did you get injured? Monkey bars. I mean…

Nine down, almost halfway. Go again, maybe make this the last set and do some non-hurty drills for a short while, before heading for netball and seeing your daughter's smile. The thought perks up your stroke and you finish with more than 20 seconds to spare. That's 20 seconds to contemplate not so much your life choices as your current choice. To quit. You ain't got much, but you've always had determination, doggedness, discipline. Grit. How would you feel about yourself if you gave up?

Get going and resolve to manage at least 20 sets. Set number 11 seems to last forever. Who knew 100 metres could be so flipping gruelling? A glance at the watch and you realise you've actually taken more than two minutes for that. Time is passing agonisingly slowly and simultaneously horribly quickly. No time to rest, got to make 12 a fast one. Only eight to go after this. Your shoulder's still hurting, but seems to be calming a little.

Seven seconds to rest this time. You begin to dread going again. What's up with you? Usually you celebrate exercise, you come through the tough times. Why is this so different? And then you realise. You're bored. BORED. BORED. BORED. The appalling fact of having to stay conscious enough to count lengths and time sets, while your mind desperately needs to wander. It's like some kind of mental torture, your brain being pulled in two opposite directions. If this were an interrogation, you would sing like a canary.

Seven seconds are up. Go again. Resent the pain in your shoulder. Resent the black line. Resent your shorts for flaring. Running shorts. Should've worn proper swim shorts. Resent your goggles. Resent the edge of the pool. Resent the Channel. Resent five more lengths. Resent 100 metres, an eternity. There are now 13 sets done, seven to go. Not sure you've got them in you and also, appallingly, know you'll definitely get through them. You had 10 seconds to rest and they're long gone. You're late for the next set. Off you go with a heavy, soul-deep sigh.

Five more lengths and you can almost see the light at the end of the tunnel. Funny how the last few sets are always the easiest, even if physically the hardest. But what's that noise behind the light at the end of the tunnel? It's nothing more than a whisper at this distance, but you know exactly what it's saying. It's reminding you of your initial plan. A hundred hundreds. Not 20. Every fibre of your being wants to finish at 20, but you know yourself well enough to know that you won't. Oh well, cross that bridge when you come to it. Time's up, off you go again.

Suddenly you remember to do that thing where you count your blessings. It's what endurance sport can teach you if you'll allow it to: how to live in gratitude. So as you swim, you give thanks for the bits of your body that don't hurt, which is all of it bar the shoulder. Almost five decades old and only ever so slightly creaky. You'll take that. And five more lengths completed. Don't bother to check how many you have left: it's either not very many at all (four) or too many to contemplate (76). Just wait for the second hand to reach the top of the dial again and away you go again.

Then something amazing happens. Somewhere along the line, literally somewhere along that black line at the bottom of the pool, you lose yourself in the act of swimming. And you realise you're revelling in your body, in your ability to push water backwards and propel yourself forwards. What an extraordinary ability humans have devised, which you're on your way to mastering.

Is this what it means to be a passenger in your own stroke? You revel in this glorious experience of being in water, in this weird and wonderful element, and owning it. Suddenly you realise you've forgotten to stop at the end of five lengths and somehow done seven. Under the circumstances, you decide to press on regardless. And that's when you recall the first time you met Duncan Goodhew. It was at a press event ahead of the London Olympics.

I can't remember what they were promoting. At the time I was presenting the BBC 5live *Breakfast Show* with the wonderful Shelagh Fogarty, another keen swimmer, and we were asked if we'd like Duncan to give us a swimming lesson, and later to race each other in the new London Aquatics Centre pool which had been freshly built for the Games. I mean...

For the lesson, we turned up to a high-end gym in the poshest bit of Kensington (which puts it quite high in the running for poshest bit of anywhere) and the 1980 Olympic breaststroke champion was waiting for us in the shallow end. The first thing he told us to do was commune with the water; to take a moment to make friends with the fact we were entering an alien environment.

Years later, I contacted Duncan to hear more about what he'd meant:

'Astronauts train in the water, because it's the closest to an off-world experience, a zero-gravity experience. We live every day standing up, sitting down, always using muscles. And so the first thing you've got to acclimatise yourself to is the fact that this stuff is supporting you. This incredible element is almost giving you an off-world experience.

'And that mutual gravity is really important, because you don't have to use any other muscles in your body, first of all.

And the second thing is that it requires a skill and it's a sense of touch. And the best thing I can compare it with is when you're playing tennis, every little angle of the racket will affect where the ball goes. Equally, as you pull or kick, every kick will have an impact on how you move in the water and how well you move through the water.

'Part and parcel of progressing in swimming is becoming more and more one with the water. So as you feel the water and touch the water, you're trying to increase your sense of touch, your sense of feel. Feel the water both with your hands and the rest of your body. So you can skim through the water as it were, or slide through the water with better efficiency and less friction.

'And also you learn how to use each part of your body in a better way to get more propulsion. So you swim faster per stroke and further per stroke. All of those elements come together to make swimming a very interesting experience and one that really, once you engage in the detail, sets it apart from every other activity you'll do.'

I went on to wonder whether Duncan took a moment to commune with the water every time he entered a pool, for every training session, every race?

'I cultivated a greater love for what I was doing, because I gave myself time and space to enjoy the experience of the water. I started to realise that if you counted lengths, the next thing you'd count was tiles. And if you swim 20,000 metres in one day, that's a heck of a lot of coloured tiles to count. So it then became, I've got to love it, I've got to love all of it.

'And coming back to what you were saying, it was the understanding of this beautiful substance that you dive into and it's such an incredible feeling as the water's rushing across your body. And the more you do it, the more sensitive your body becomes to that feeling. People ask me, is there a difference between types of water? It's like pillows. Is there a difference between pillows when you sleep on them? There are soft pillows and hard pillows, and likewise each pool feels slightly different. And that sensitivity actually made everything beautiful.'

Back in the 20-metre pool in Raynes Park, something strange and utterly wonderful is happening to me. I don't realise it at the time, because everything becomes a bit of a blur. The thick black line at the bottom of the pool, the swim stroke, arm, catch, kick, breathe left, breathe right, the endless tumble turns... I don't just lose track of lengths. And I don't just lose track of time. I lose track of everything.

The best way I can think to describe it is I transcend. I'm dimly aware of my body swimming up and down the pool – the black line, the stroke, the breaths, the turns – but I'm watching from a great height. I don't feel or think anything. It's neither great joy nor anything remotely like sadness. It's pure contentment. Elsewhere in the pool, Eeyore is fretting, Piglet hesitating, Rabbit calculating, Owl pontificating. And I'm Pooh. I simply am.

I'd love to write thousands of words about this, but I sense they don't exist. I'd love to know how to return to that state. I'd love to teach people to get there. Impossible. That's the point, I suppose. Though the 13th-century Persian poet Rumi has a good go:

There's a field beyond right and wrong
And I'll meet you there.
In this field the soul rests on the grass
And the world is too full for mere words
And the phrase 'each other' just doesn't
make any sense.

I become a little obsessed. Is this what happens when you master meditation? I've tried loads of meditation and never reached anywhere near the transcendence of that Saturday morning in the pool; the state of simply being, like Winnie the Pooh, or Rumi's field beyond right and wrong. Duncan expressed it like this:

> 'Swimming can really put you in the moment. If you want to use pool swimming for meditation purposes, then you can do that. You know how many strokes per length, you know what time you do. There's a great rhythm to it. It's such a controlled box, a swimming pool, which plays very well to certain moods. Vassos, you've always been known as a runner, haven't you, so swimming is where yoga meets running really. It's got that whole zen to it, a meditative process, as well as being a skill sport, too.'

Time has no meaning as I continue up and down the pool. Up and down, up and down, in the greatest of flow states. An elite ultra runner, bestselling author and smash hit podcaster. Rich Roll started out as a competitive swimmer:

> 'There's something really unique about swimming, because you're stripped of all external stimuli other than the black line at the bottom of the pool. That allows time to bend in a weird way and you're just taken to another place. It is a form of meditation and there is a self-transcendence aspect to it, especially when you're putting in tons of volume and gigantic distances, where you're just meeting yourself in a really special place that the modern world doesn't really afford us, unless we get out of our comfort zone and explore what those possibilities are.
>
> 'So 100%, I totally agree. There's something really unique about that experience which allows you to learn about

yourself. There's a lot of talk in ultra running about a similar thing, but you're in nature and there's a different natural aspect to that experience that lends itself to some form of self-transcendence. But this is what happens when you take away all of that, and there's absolutely nothing to distract you other than your own mind and body.'

After a few hours, or perhaps a few days, or maybe a few minutes, I come back to myself. My shoulder starts hurting again. I notice other people in the pool. I realise I've had some kind of out-of-body experience, but I'm completely calm; not remotely worried that I might have looked odd or been doing anything embarrassing.

I reach the end of the pool and pause. Look at the watch. I've been going for over three and a half hours and swum almost 11 kilometres. I have no desire to leave the pool. I want to get back into flow. I swim on, being careful to notice the last things I remembered noticing. The black line, the long, languid strokes, the side-to-side breathing (was it something to do with the two hemispheres of the brain?), the tumble turns.

I keep at it for over half an hour, attempting to conjure transcendence. While I'm calm throughout, I'm also disappointingly aware of everything around me. Other swimmers, the weather, my shoulder, the passage of time. Four hours after starting my swim, I call it a day. A seminal, spiritual, seismic day.

I never did take my daughter to netball.

11

Swimming History

Everyone should have heard of Gertrude Ederle. She changed the world. And everyone should have heard of Lynne Cox. She saved the world.

Today, many people *have* heard of Gertrude Ederle, thanks to the brilliant film *Young Woman and the Sea*. In case you haven't, firstly please watch it. It's ace. And secondly, she truly was amazing.

She was born in New York in 1905, the daughter of an immigrant German butcher. Money was scarce and young Trudy's social standing was hardly high. Her immigrant roots did her no favours and neither did her gender. At the time, women didn't really 'do' sport. It was considered unseemly. Not to mention too much for their supposedly fragile bodies to bear. As for swimming? Forget it – that was unsuitable, unbecoming, unbefitting, in very poor taste.

Ederle didn't care about any of that. She'd survived measles as a child despite a dire diagnosis from the local doctor and thought nothing of challenging social norms. She was also expected to agree to an arranged marriage and wanted nothing to do with that either. Her mum was very much on her side, though, and with her support she learned to swim in New Jersey, joining a newly-formed women's swim club.

She was also lucky that her Italian-born trainer, Louis de Breda Handley, literally wrote the book on the front crawl (or American crawl as it was known at the time). When *Encyclopaedia Britannica* needed an entry dedicated to swimming, they asked Handley to author it and under his guidance Trudy developed into an excellent swimmer. She would always say that she was 'happiest between the waves'. And young Trudy found she didn't just enjoy swimming, she was also so good at it she was chosen to represent the USA at the 1924 Summer Olympics in Paris, and won two individual bronze medals and a relay gold.

At the time, the world's greatest endurance challenge was swimming the English Channel. Only five people had managed it since Captain Matthew Webb's first successful crossing in 1875. Webb instantly became a huge celebrity and basked in the international adulation. He wrote a book called *The Art of Swimming*, which you can still buy on eBay. He then did the full megastar thing and started giving product endorsements. Within months you could buy Captain Matthew Webb pottery and use Captain Matthew Webb matches to light your candles.

News of his feat travelled fast and soon he was journeying around the world doing swimming exhibitions. Fatally, he started believing his own hype. In 1883 he decided to become the first person to tackle the dangerous Whirlpool Rapids at the bottom of Niagara Falls and drowned. It took four days to recover his body. Today in Dover, there's a statue of Webb looking out across the Channel towards France. And in his hometown of Dawley in Shropshire there's a memorial with the inscription 'Nothing great is easy.'

By 1925, the people who had successfully swum the Channel had all been men. In fact, it was widely believed that women were simply not capable of achieving any feat of endurance, let alone the toughest one on earth. Yeah, shut up, said Gertrude Ederle (or the 1920s equivalent). Despite the social and financial pressures she had to contend with, she decided to become the first – and to prove a point in the process.

The only thing was, her new coach, Jabez Wolffe from Scotland, was now actively working against her. He had tried and failed to swim the Channel 22 times, and as a result had no interest in seeing a woman succeed. It would make him look bad by comparison. So during her first attempt in 1925, while Gertrude was having a quick rest, he claimed he thought she was drowning, reached out from the support boat and touched her, instantly disqualifying her.

Trudy was outraged, but no quitter. She returned the following year, now aged 20, with a different coach, TW Burgess, a maverick water polo Olympic medallist and the second person to successfully swim the Channel. He promised he'd only pull Ederle out of the water if she asked.

At 7.08 a.m. on 6 August 1926, smothered in mutton grease for warmth and wearing what was considered a risqué two-piece bathing suit she'd designed herself, Trudy Ederle waded into the choppy waters at Cap Gris-Nez in France. This time the weather, rather than her coach, conspired against her. The wind blew up, waves grew larger and ferries were cancelled. Members of the press in a following boat started throwing up into the water. She also had to contend with vicious cross tides, floating debris and poisonous jellyfish. But she kept going.

After 14 hours and 31 minutes in the wild, cold sea, Gertrude Ederle landed on the Kent coast at Kingstown. She became the first woman – and sixth person overall – to swim the Channel. She broke the previous fastest time by two hours. Her new record lasted for a generation. Fame was instant (although the first person to greet her on British soil was a customs officer demanding to see her passport).

When Trudy returned to New York, over two million people lined the streets for a ticker tape parade to celebrate her. It remains the biggest sporting parade in history. The *New*

York Times described her achievement as 'the biggest thing in athletics ever done by a woman, or a man for that matter.' She met the president and was paid thousands to appear at Brooklyn's Strand Theatre. She toured the country in vaudeville shows and even had a dance step named after her. For a time, she was a bigger deal than Babe Ruth.

The Great Depression put an end to the shows, and then in 1933 Ederle fell down the steps in her apartment building and twisted her spine. It left her bedridden for years and she didn't make another public appearance until the World's Fair in New York in 1939. She'd had poor hearing since childhood due to the measles and by the 1940s was almost completely deaf. She spent her later decades teaching swimming to deaf children. She had many offers of marriage and refused them all. She died in 2003 aged 98.

Gertrude Ederle inspired women everywhere. Suddenly sport wasn't potentially just a male preserve. Suddenly women realised they could take on whatever challenges they wanted and do so every bit as well as men – if not better. Of course, the world has taken its time catching up, and women are still struggling to be taken as seriously and paid the same as men, but Gertrude Ederle began that journey. Gertrude Ederle changed the world.

Lynne Cox saved the world.

I had the great honour of interviewing her at some length and somebody should make a film about Lynne, too.

In 1987, at the height of the Cold War, she became the first person to swim the Bering Strait. She set off in freezing water from the island of Little Diomede in Alaska, and just over two miles and two hours later, she arrived on Big Diomede, then in the Soviet Union – a short way on the map, but a mighty distance in terms of bridging worlds.

Weeks later at the White House, U.S. President Ronald Reagan and Soviet leader Mikhail Gorbachev signed the

Intermediate Range Nuclear Forces Treaty signifying the beginning of the end of the Cold War. Reagan and Gorbachev raised their glasses and the Russian made a toast:

'It took one brave American by the name of Lynne Cox just two hours to swim from one of our countries to the other. We saw on television how sincere and friendly the meeting was between our people and the Americans when she stepped on to the Soviet shore. She proved by her courage how close to each other our peoples live.'

Lynne Cox dived into icy water and literally thawed the Cold War. I think that's simply epic and even more so when you find out how long the swim was in gestation. I was so excited to ask her about it.

'It took 11 years to get permission to do it. Actually, when I proposed doing the swim, it was during the height of the Cold War. So people thought it was absolutely crazy, because relations between our two countries were so strained. But I think that there has to be this idea that you can make a difference, that you can make a positive difference, and you just keep working toward it and then at some point things shift.

'After I decided to try to get permission and then train for it, it became an all-consuming activity. I mean, I was working on it every single day for those 11 years, trying to figure out how to get permission, trying to figure out who I'd get for the support team, where we would start, what the currents would be, how to fund it, who would come along as the medical support. It was a huge project.

'And after seven or eight or nine or 10 years, I wasn't willing to give up on it, because I felt that we really needed to figure out how the United States and Soviet Union could diminish tensions and look at each other as neighbours and even as friends. I realised that we needed to have a change in the world. We needed to figure out how to get along.'

Lynne was already a hugely accomplished swimmer. In 1971 she was among the first group of teenagers to complete the crossing of the Catalina Island channel in California. She had twice held the record for the fastest crossing of the English Channel (9 hours 57 minutes in 1972 and 9 hours 36 minutes in 1973). In 1975, she became the first woman to swim the 10-mile Cook Strait in New Zealand, and the following year was the first person to swim both the Straits of Magellan in Chile and around the Cape of Good Hope in South Africa.

But the Bering Strait was a whole new level. It was a lovely idea – swim from one superpower to another to show how close they really are – but the reality was an almost impossible list of questions and problems. This was long pre-internet, and answers came painfully slowly. For instance, Lynne had no way of knowing what the water temperature would be, which is kind of key.

It took two years of writing letters to Alaska's Department of Fish and Game to get the answer: around 6 or 7 degrees Celsius. The next question was whether she would be able to cope in those temperatures for an extended period of time:

'Because of that, I reached out to Dr Keating at the University of London, who was the world's expert in hypothermia, and we had years of correspondence in figuring out how could I survive or do well in the cold. I did that with all sorts of people to try to get permission to swim the Bering Strait. This was a huge puzzle. It was intriguing.

'How do you get all these different parts to come together? How do you get the political permission to do it? How do you get the support team to come and support the swim? How do you swim in water that cold? How do you fund this?

How do you get to Little Diomede, Alaska? So much to learn. And back then there wasn't the internet. Much of it was done by letter and telex and eventually fax. So lots of time went by before I would receive any responses.'

Eventually, after more than a decade putting together the pieces of the giant logistical jigsaw, Lynne and her team could set off, thanks to free tickets from Alaska Airways. She arrived on Little Diomede, but with 30 hours to go until her planned set off time, still hadn't heard from the Soviets. Instead, two Soviet military ships appeared in the middle of the strait, to which the US responded by sending jet fighters. For a short while it looked like her peace mission was backfiring spectacularly. But with 24 hours to go, word finally came through from President Gorbachev. The swim was on! Equally excited were the indigenous Iñupiaq Alaska Natives, who were to join the swim in their traditional skin boats and see their relatives on the Russian side for the first time in decades.

For more than 40 years, the 2.7 miles between the Diomede Islands was nicknamed the 'Ice Curtain'. The International Date Line also runs through the Bering Strait and it is literally a different day on either side of it (well, not quite, because of local time zones, but almost). For more than 40 years ordinary citizens of both countries were not allowed on the shores of Big Diomede. The Soviets turned it into a military base. Native Iñupiaq people who'd been hunting, fishing and moving freely between the islands for thousands of years were stripped of their lands and traditions. And the Soviets were extremely reluctant to reopen that particular border.

But Lynne Cox is special. Who else would have had the tenacity to keep asking for permission for 11 long years? She wrote to four Soviet leaders: Brezhnev, Andropov, Chernenko and finally Gorbachev, who replied. And, frankly, who else could have pulled off the swim? For a start, Lynne has something almost unique called neutral buoyancy. A research physiologist at the University of California in Santa Barbara once told her: 'Your proportion of fat to muscle is perfectly balanced so you don't float or sink in the water; you're at one with the water. We've never seen anything like this before.' Almost all of the rest of us either sink in water (negative buoyancy) or float (positive buoyancy).

She also has a superhuman ability to resist cold. Even during those long hours between Alaska and Siberia, even as she watched her limbs go blue and splotchy, her body had this astonishing ability to redirect its heat to the vital organs of her brain, chest and abdomen. This allowed her to keep pushing forward. She knew from long hours in the English Channel that she could tolerate cold water. After all, she'd held that record for the fastest crossing between England and France not once but twice. But this was different gravy. Nothing could prepare her for this.

Lynne entered the water on the morning of 7 August 1987. It was foggy. The cold was worse than she'd ever imagined. She recalls, 'It was like a vampire pulling the heat from my body. I looked down at my fingers and they were totally grey, like the hands of a cadaver.' And then she became lost in the fog.

Her guides had obviously never made the journey before and feared they'd miss their target of Big Diomede. And then in what Lynne describes as 'one of the most beautiful sights of my life,' a Russian ship emerged from the fog and showed them the way. The swim would be complete when Lynne touched a rock out at sea, the closest piece of Soviet soil. But mid-swim she was informed that a welcoming party had gathered on the beach half a mile further on. The concern was that another half mile in the icy waters could kill her. She had a decision to make.

She says, 'I decided to go that extra half mile, because I felt like if I touch rock, instead of somebody's hand, what have I done? Nothing! There was no connection with the people on the opposite shore.' After two hours and seven minutes in the deathly water, she arrived to great cheers on the beach. The Soviets had sent a welcome party and two Russian soldiers helped her to her feet. And that's when Lynne accidentally asked for a granny:

> 'I instantly felt this heat from their warm hands. And they were speaking Russian and I thought, oh my gosh, we really made it! Actually, I really meant to ask for a shawl because I felt that that symbolised the warmth of the Soviet people. But instead I used the word "babushka", which means granny – and it turns out that they actually did have a grandmother on the beach for me. She was one of the medical doctors who was there to make sure that I was okay after the swim. So instead of having a shawl giving me warmth at the end of the swim, she was leaning on me and giving me her body heat.
>
> 'But those moments are so special, because it's that human connection of realising that we grew up in different worlds and different cultures, but we're all human beings, and we all laugh and cry, and hope and dream, and have sad moments, and believe in things that can be done. And I think that's what's so important – that we realise we have a lot of the same language inside us.'

These days Lynne lives in Southern California, where she still swims every day, as well as giving inspirational talks and writing books for both adults and children. Nine books now and counting. And she travels with her husband who works with symphony orchestras all over the United States. But there's always swimming:

> 'Well, actually, I like to be alone with my thoughts for long stretches of time. I like to read and then have something to

think about. Or consider what I'm doing in my life, and what I want to be doing and how to get there.

'Swimming in the open water is a time where you're watching the sunrise, and the pelicans and seals glide by, and the people on their outrigger canoes. And you're out there enjoying being in the vast ocean versus being in a small cubbyhole of a room. It's a time to think about things.

'There's no cell phone. There's no computer. There's no one knocking on your door. It's just you thinking. There are times where you get tired or hungry, where you get cold and you want to stop, and you have to talk yourself into it – okay, just swim another quarter mile or another 200 metres – so that's all I do and it's really worked out well!'

'It's really worked out well!' Might just be one of the great understatements.

12

Swimming Downhill IV

I bounce into my next lesson with Ray desperate to show off how much work I've done. How committed I've been to the drills. I've got it, I'm sure I have. I abandoned my family for large parts of our once-in-a-lifetime winter sun holiday just to perfect a drill called catch-catch-elbow pause. Twice a day, without fail, every day of our holiday, including Christmas Day and Caroline's birthday. I was even in the sea on the day the news came through of our beloved Labrador Holly's sudden passing.

I'd sauntered into the hotel's reception area after yet another session of Indian Ocean swim drills to find the four other members of my family huddled round a table in floods of tears. Our youngest daughter was wailing loudly. Hotel staff were looking concerned, while desperately trying to usher them away from where other families were checking in for their own once-in-a-lifetime holidays.

Imagine the first thing you see when you arrive in paradise is a family weeping inconsolably. They must have been wondering what they'd let themselves in for. As for me, I felt somehow that I'd let everyone down by being absent when the news came through. But perhaps it was worth the sacrifices. When I commit, I properly commit.

I had put the work in, and I was excited to return to Ray and be told how well I'd done. I was eager to start finding out exactly what 'swimming downhill' feels like. I was disappointed on both counts. I think the best way to relay what happened next is via the email Ray sent me the day after our lesson.

From: Ray Gibbs
To: Vassos Alexander
Cc: Clare
Date: 5 January 2024 at 20:51
Subject: Chin Up Sunshine!

Hi Vassos,

I couldn't help noticing that you were a bit deflated as you left my unit on Thursday. You absolutely shouldn't be!

Your stroke has changed for the better (watch/listen to the 'first swim' file), because you have been repeating the correct movement (when performing the catch-catch). Okay, you didn't nail the 'switch' element of the drill, but you will.

You also mentioned that you're worried about 'getting it wrong again' between lessons. If you still feel that way, please reply to Clare (cc'd) as the tube strike has opened up a couple of slots.

Ray

Describing my mood after the lesson as 'a bit deflated' isn't quite accurate. I was proper gutted. I sulked for two whole days. To hell with swimming! But then, on the Saturday afternoon 48 hours after finding out I'd been doing my drills wrong, I head to the pool to keep practising. Perhaps I'll never get this right, I think. Perhaps the Channel is too big a challenge. But one thing's for certain. It won't be for lack of effort. I haven't come this far just to come this far.

I refocus. I reframe the drills as things I *get* to do, rather than things I've *got* to do. And it works. Slowly, slowly, things begin to click underwater. I experience a fleeting sensation of what it must be like to swim correctly. And then it happens again. And again. The feeling becomes more regular and more attainable.

Praise duly comes from Ray and the drills become more and more complicated. I especially enjoy the fortnight when I get to swim half a length staccato – exaggerating every movement and pausing after each one – then transition into the normal stroke over the remainder of the length. It's the aquatic equivalent of doing strides to improve your running. The second half of those lengths feels powerful, easy, fast, effortless, fun. Swimming downhill!

No wonder Ray came so highly recommended. I was still far from perfect (still am, as a matter of fact), but I could sense the progress and, more importantly, I was beginning to viscerally understand where the process was taking me. It was a real buzz. It's why he became a teacher in the first place, because Ray feels the same excitement whenever one of his students finally makes the breakthrough:

'Hairs are standing up on my arm, because it's such a great thing to be able to give to people. That's a really special moment in swimming. But you have to practise to get it. If you don't put in the hours that you did, then you don't get that, unless you're very, very lucky and you've got naturally excellent technique, but those people are few and far between.'

Ray's journey to the unprepossessing commercial unit in Canary Wharf, where he's solidly booked for months in advance, is interesting to say the least. It takes in the early, exciting days of triathlon, when the sport was new, as well as the centuries-old warehouses and 'geezers' of the East End of London:

'I took up swimming when I took up triathlon in my late 20s. You've obviously got to be able to swim to do triathlon and I joined the Masters swim club, because back then triathlon was a real minority sport. My British Triathlon Federation membership number was 289, so there were 288 people in the country doing triathlon before me, if you can imagine that.

'There wasn't really any triathlon club, so I joined the Masters club, which is basically for ex-swimmers to carry on swimming once they've given up club swimming. But all that did, because they were mainly sprinters, was make me into a sprinter and I became a pretty good 100-metre swimmer, but I wanted to do triathlons, which take two, two and a half hours.

'So then I had to start looking at the stroke and looking at the technique, figuring out how these long-distance swimmers were able to maintain it. But no one was doing that at the time. Well, no one who could make a living out of it. There were only 289 people doing triathlon. You could go to your local leisure centre if you were lucky and learn to swim as an adult from zero. And there was Masters swim for already amazing swimmers, who actually don't know that much about technique because they're natural swimmers. But nobody like me to tell people, so I had to figure it out for myself.

'And that really helps me as a teacher, because I've been through that process. And for me, it was a more painful process, if you can believe it, because that's all figured out now. I was pre-internet, so there were no videos to watch.

'And so I figured it out and I ended up being a pretty good swimmer for triathlon. I used to come out in the top five or six at most races. And then friends started asking me "How did you do that? Because we're stuck. We put in loads of effort and we're stuck." So I started helping friends and I did a little bit of swimming teaching with kids as well.

'At the same time I was running one of the huge antiques warehouses in Bermondsey, South East London. What that gave me was an amazing eye for detail, because you live and die by detail if you're dealing in that sort of thing. Something could be worthless or it can be worth a great deal. It's all down to the detail. Cracks, bends, woodworm, you name it.

'So often when I say to people that's what I did before this, they say, "Well, you couldn't think of anything more different," but they're wrong, because my job's all about detail. All my life, I've been a details guy. I have to wear glasses now, but I still have to spot the detail.

'So then that job changed, because Bermondsey stopped being cheap property full of warehouses to being extremely expensive, actually. All the warehouses got bought up by property developers and so I was at a point where I thought, "Okay, what am I going to do with my life?" And my dad died around about that time and it gives me a bit of a wake-up call. And you think to yourself, "Okay, right, life's short. What do I enjoy doing?"

'I had a few quid, not much, and one of my friends had a bike shop in one of the units in Canary Wharf. And I thought, "Well, this would make a really good place for an endless pool, and we'll rig it up with the cameras. You can see what you can never see in a public swimming pool or even a private swimming pool." So I took the plunge. I emptied the bank account, built the pool, built the changing rooms, built everything.

'I was very lucky, because the triathlon thing went crazy pretty much from when I opened. Then this ball started rolling about open water swimming. And ex-swimmers started going back into open water. So I was always busy. And I love it. Oh my goodness, yeah. Speak to any teacher. Teaching someone who wants to learn is the greatest job in the world.'

13

Swimming Serpentine

One evening on holiday, in a village market in the south of France, I paid €10 for a framed, personalised caricature of our family, which I thought we'd throw away as soon as we got home, but which has stood proudly on our breakfast bar ever since and makes us all smile every time we look at it.

When our Swedish neighbour Hans sold his original shares in Spotify and moved out of Barnes to buy a small country or two, he asked if we wanted his spring-free trampoline for a good price. It's big, this trampoline; massive, far too big for our garden, with multiple bounce zones. It would have cost hundreds of pounds when Hans bought it a matter of months previously. He gave it to us for £50 and all three of our kids (and all of their friends) have spent much of their childhoods bouncing ever since.

Throughout the 15 years since the arrival of our first puppy, Holly, our house has smelt of wet Labrador. We've long since become so used to the pong that we no longer notice and guests are always too polite to mention. One Christmas morning, our teenage son found a £17 oil diffuser in his stocking. His room smelt significantly worse than wet Labrador, but he didn't seem to want to use the new present. It soon found its way to our hallway and suddenly we would open our front door to the aromas of lemongrass, rosemary, lavender... And everyone started telling us how fragrant our house smelt.

Three of our finest examples of money well spent (that final one down to Santa, of course). But the best value of all is the £20 that leaves my account every 1 January. I defy you to spend a better £20 than the annual membership of the Serpentine Swim Club. For less than the cost of three pints in any of the pubs within a two-mile radius, you get to swim in a glorious lake in the centre of London, every day of the year.

The Serpentine was created in 1730 on the orders of Queen Caroline, wife of King George II. One of the first artificial lakes in the world designed to appear natural, it stretches for about a mile from east to west in a graceful, 'serpentine' curve. On the southern shore, there's a free art gallery of the same name, as well as a cafe with tables arranged along the water's edge. Runners and walkers enjoy a wide sandstone path around the lake, 2.5 miles in circumference, while tourists hire pedalos from the north-east edge. There are reeds along some of the shoreline, but mostly the path slopes gently directly down to the water.

The lake is particularly renowned for its resident population of swans gliding regally across the surface, as well as its numerous ducks, geese and moorhens. Grebes can sometimes be spotted diving beneath the surface. Coots make their nests among the buoys of the cordoned-off swimming area near the cafe. There are fish under the surface though they remain more elusive. Queen Caroline knew what she was doing. The Serpentine retains a sense of serene seclusion, offering a peaceful respite amidst the bustle of central London.

Members' swim times are 5 a.m. to 9.30 a.m. and in the summer it becomes a public lido from 10 a.m. Members can also enter the famous Saturday morning races, which are taken simultaneously very seriously, and not seriously at all. They tend to be handicapped, with the strongest swimmers starting last. And if you fancy seeing your picture in the newspapers, just turn up and swim on Christmas Day and/or New Year's Day, when there's bound to be a press photographer on hand to capture an image of 'Hardy winter swimmers' for their news desk.

The Serpentine is a detour of approximately 50 metres on my cycle to work. If I'm in the water by 5:15 a.m., I can have a decent swim and still make it on time to the Virgin Radio *Breakfast Show*, on air at 6.30 a.m. You tend to have the lake to yourself at 5 a.m., though not always. I've still made several friends among the happy, early morning community who arrive soon after me. Mark the barrister usually swims at 6 a.m. but comes earlier if he has a case outside London. Xavier the teacher has a wonderful way about him and a French accent straight out of central casting. Jimmy dives in wearing the shorts of his beloved Leyton Orient, often enjoys a drink with the retired Bishop of London, and walks to his dawn swim from his grace-and-favour flat in swanky nearby Knightsbridge. Desmond is a Member of Parliament and former government minister. And often arriving as early if not earlier than I do, the senior quartet includes Ani, the tiny force of nature who once forced a group of young men to return a stolen bike just by looking at them, and Mary with the gorgeous, blind, black Labrador.

Sometimes, when it's dark and deserted and I'm sure I'm alone, I'll treat myself to a sneaky skinny dip. I'll change by the side of the lake, rather than the changing room, and enter the water by the bannister in the middle of the swimming area, which is furthest away from either entry gate. I'll only whip off my shorts after a final, furtive double-check that nobody's about. Then it's swiftly into the water where nobody can see your naked bottom.

There's something magical about nude swimming, all the more so in the centre of London. Being submerged in nature and your birthday suit in an urban environment gives a wonderful feeling of freedom, to the extent that my watch and wedding ring feel like they're spoiling the purity of the experience, and I'll take them off, too. I did once lose my wedding ring in this manner, accidentally dropping it in the water never to be seen again. (I subsequently lost its replacement while swimming in Vietnam, and a third wedding ring in the North Sea in Whitstable. The cold water shrinks fingers and rings fall off unnoticed. It's a good job Caroline and I aren't precious about them.)

I especially love the Serpentine in winter. The va-va-voom from the cold water springboards me into the rest of my day. Once, the week before Christmas on the final day of a fortnight-long, UK-wide Big Freeze, I arrived to find the lake frozen solid. Unusually, two people were there before me – probably something to do with the lure of breaking the ice to get into water, which is about as cold as it gets.

Until that day, in the five years I'd been open water swimming I'd never experienced water below 1 degree. The lowest so far was 1.8 degrees during lockdown. At that time, the Serpentine was closed and we discovered the joys and freedom of swimming in the River Thames. Just west of Teddington Lock was our wild swimming haven, and one day the Lock froze over as the temperatures plummeted. Our trusty food thermometer doubles pretty well as a cold water gauge and our little swimming posse were all thrilled as the readout showed the water had fallen below 2 degrees for the first time ever.

Open water swimmers can become a little obsessed with water temperatures in winter. The sea around the UK will always be warmest, getting down to 6 or sometimes 5 degrees. The rivers are colder, often 3 degrees, sometimes 2 and, as I say, once the Thames was 1.8 just west of the frozen Teddington Lock. And the lakes get coldest of all.

This particular pre-Christmas morning, the three of us tried unsuccessfully to break the ice at the Serpentine's edge. Too thick. I wandered to the club's somewhat spartan changing room (small room nearby with some benches, hooks, a loo and a kettle) and retrieved an umbrella from lost property. I took it to the end of the pontoon and had a smash at the ice in the middle of the lake with the handle. It cracked, then broke (fortunately the ice, not the brolly). I undressed and quickly climbed straight down the ladder into the water. No time for second thoughts, plus I was keen to be the first one in on this auspicious, ice-covered day. Pathetic, I know, but you would, wouldn't you? It's like making the first footprints in fresh snow.

We measured the temperature later – 0.7 degrees. I can't honestly tell you it feels much different from 1.8 or even 3 degrees, but it does feel magical getting in among the ice. I splashed about, breaking more ice, until there was around 20 metres of water available for swimming. I didn't stay in the water longer than four or five minutes. The rule of thumb is 'max double the degrees in minutes', so 5 degrees, maximum 10 minutes, and so on, which I tend to push the limits of. Unwisely in this case. After I got myself out, dried and dressed, watching the others in the water made me want to go in again, so I did, for another four or five minutes.

Then the cycle on to work with freezing hands, ears, feet… Always a hell of a struggle. I was cycling down Constitution Hill towards Buckingham Palace with frozen fingers necessarily covering bike brakes and feeling like they might implode with cold. But then I arrived at work with ALL the endorphins.

On the way to the Serpentine that morning, I'd felt an illness coming on, lurking around the edges of my eyes and throat. The cold water would boost my immune system, I'd decided. Head the lurgy off at the pass. It had worked in the past, but, it turns out, there are limits, and somewhere along the pontoon and splashing in the icy water that morning, I'd crossed them. The following two days were spent in bed with full-on man flu – the first time in over a year I'd been forced to miss my daily exercise. I did try to go for a gentle run, just to keep the streak going, but even I could tell I needed to succumb to the body's desperate need to rest and recover.

It's interesting, though. Exactly how much cold water is good for you and what are the limits? Why does the cold water feel easier on some days than others? Do you really need a layer of brown fat to spend any length of time in cold water? Why does cold water feel so much colder than cold air?[1] And at the extreme end of all this, how bloody hard is an ice mile?

An ice mile is swimming a full mile in water 5 degrees or below, wearing nothing but a standard costume, goggles and a single swim hat. Despite all the winter swimming I've done over the past few years, despite the ice bath in my back garden, I'm nowhere near. When the water falls below 5 degrees, I struggle to make it even a quarter of a mile or two laps of the Serpentine swim zone. Usually one lap. If you're being kind, you could put it down to the fact that I'm skinnier than your average open water swimmer. But then, kind reader, you'd better not meet Calum Hudson of the Wild Swimming Brothers (the middle one) who achieved an ice mile in a lido in Brixton and looks as svelte as Michael Phelps:

'It was a dream I was chasing maybe four years. Gradually building up. I started in exactly the same place as you are, thinking how does everybody go over 400 metres, let alone a kilometre, let alone the mile. And my journey has been that journey right from the beginning.

[1] I once paid a small fortune for a session in a cryotherapy chamber set at -140 degrees Celsius. It wasn't exactly easy, but it wasn't far off being easy. Compared to cold water, cold air can't lay a glove on you. This is because water is much better at conducting heat than air. So when you're submerged in cold water, it quickly draws a ton of heat from your skin, making you feel much colder than in much colder air.

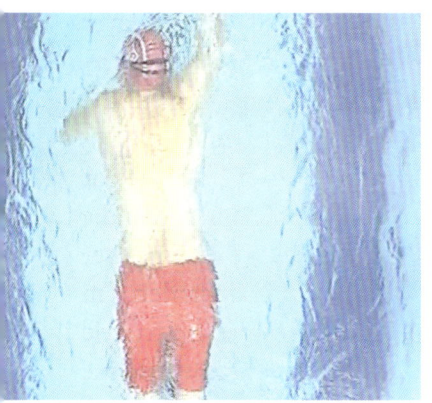
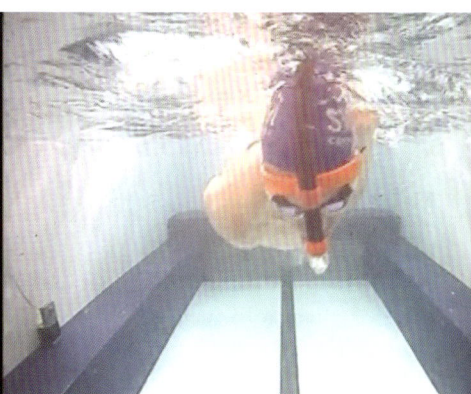

⌃ Learning to 'swim downhill' in a tank in east London.

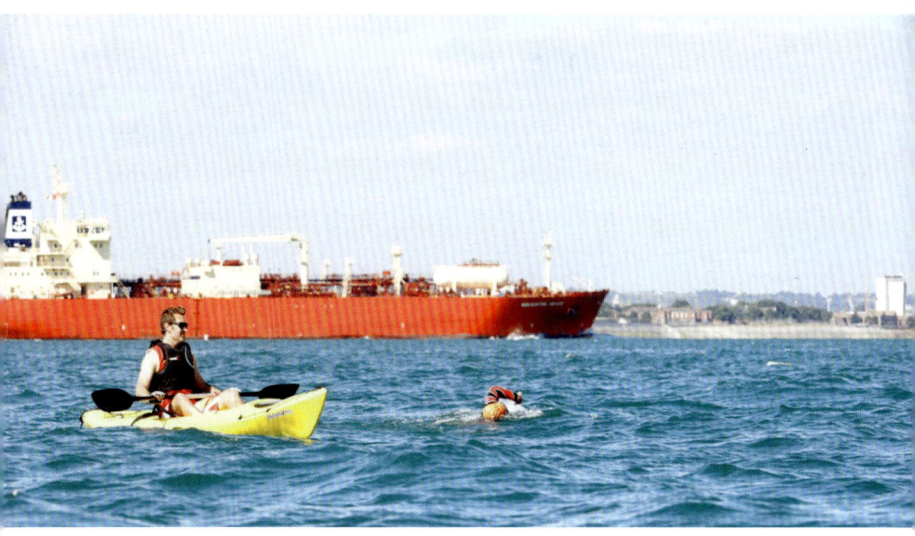

⌃ First long swim, Portsmouth to Isle of Wight dodging jellyfish, ferries and oil tankers... I was hooked!

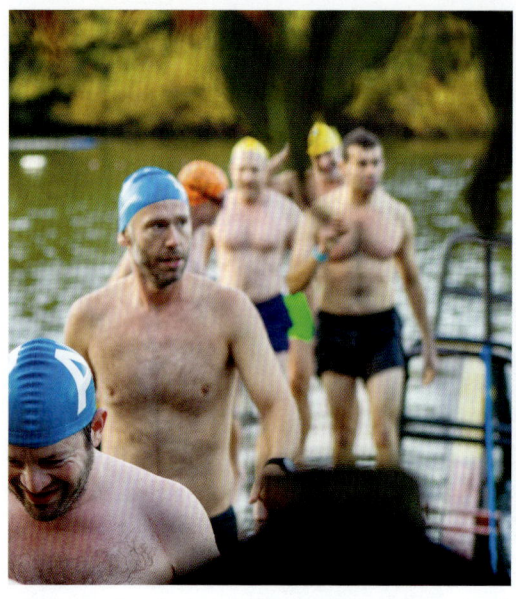
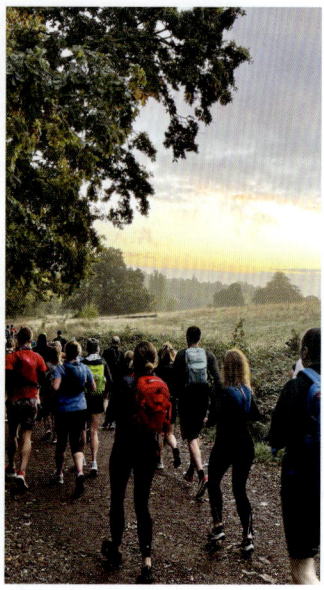

⚆ Swimming the length of London from Hampstead to Brixton… *The Swimmer, London* is just ace!

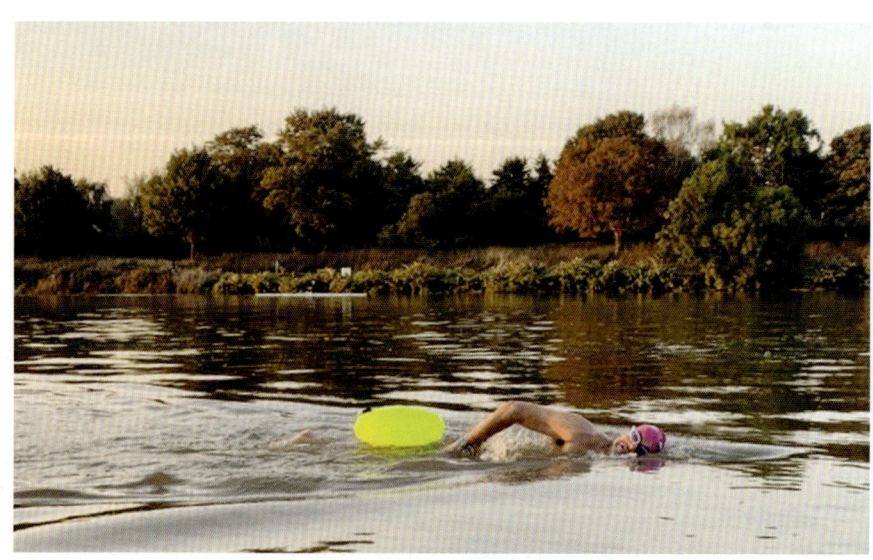

⚆ Training swim in the Thames.

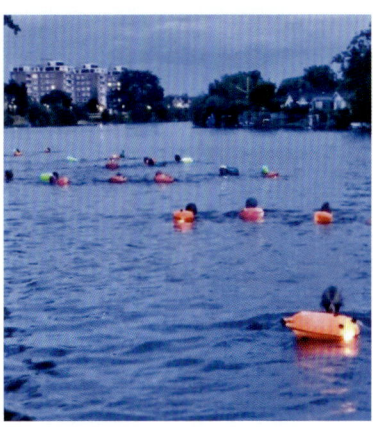

≫ Night swimming in the Thames.

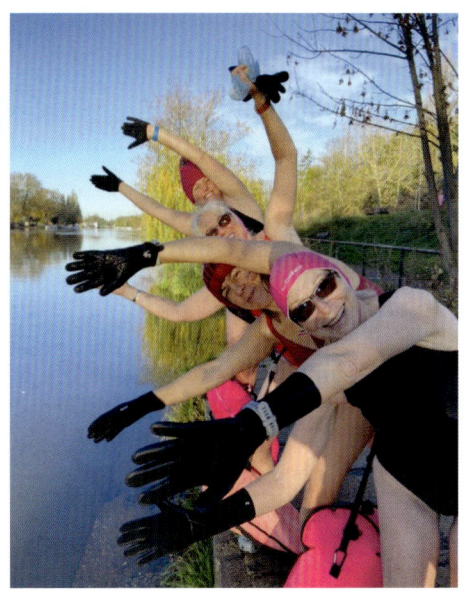

≫ Teddington Bluetits preparing for a winter swim.

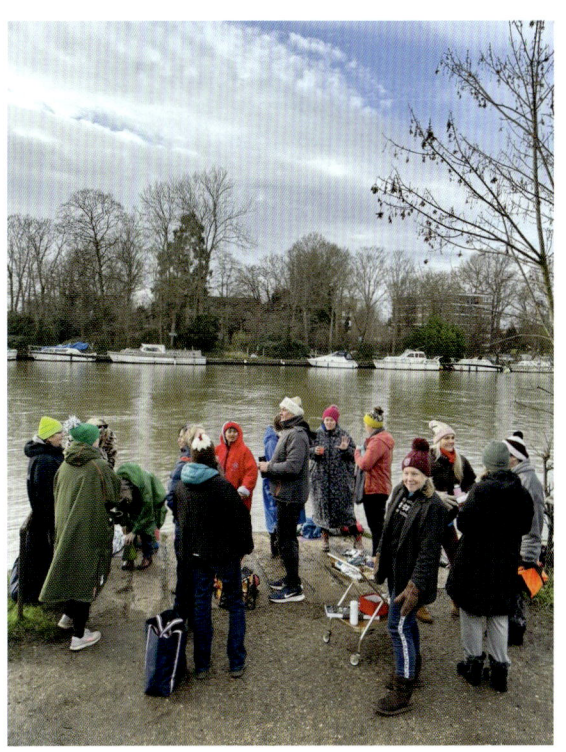

≪ Lakes, drakes, cakes and bakes… Marlene with her famous trolley and the traditional Bluetits debrief.

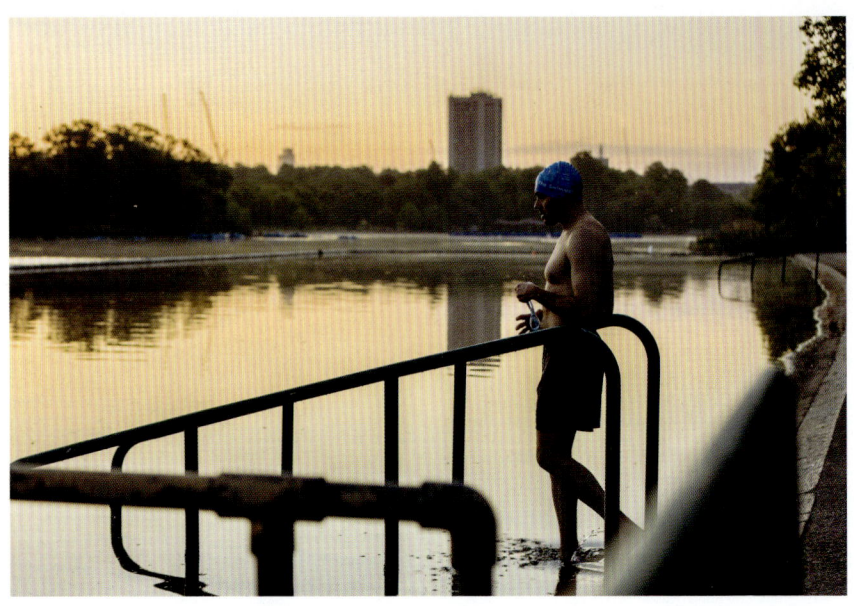

⌃ Happy place. Daily dawn swim in the Serpentine on the way to work.

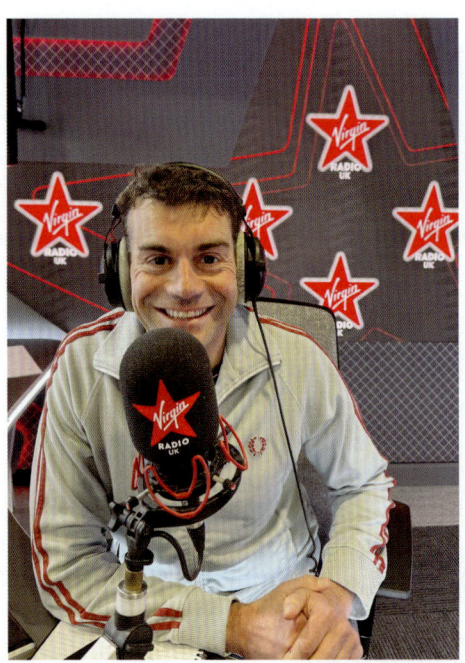

⌃ 6:30am and I've already cycled across London and swum in the Serpentine.

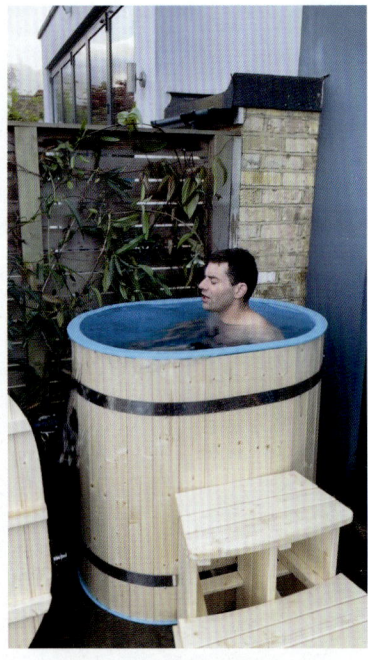

⌃ Happy-ish place: ice bath in the garden set at 2°C. Objectively horrific, but also euphoric!

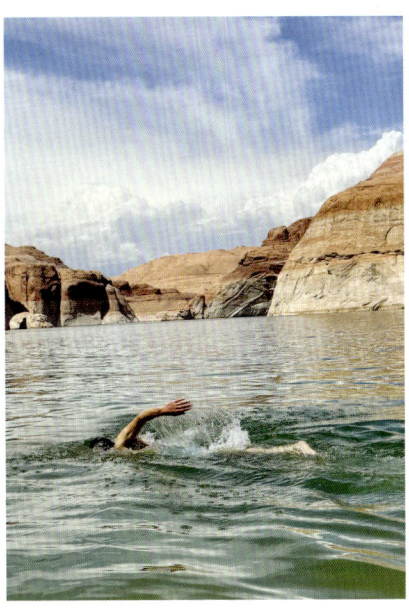

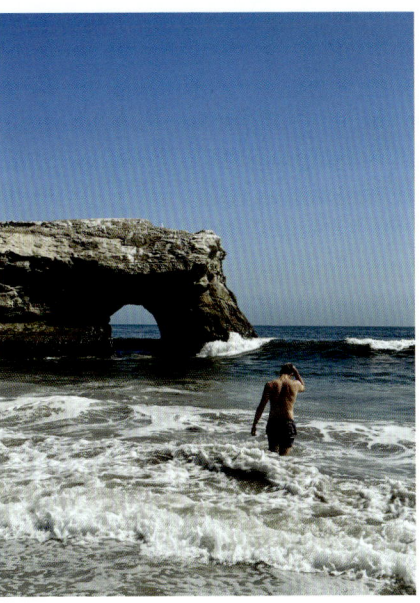

⌃ Swimming USA! What a treat to test my newfound swim stroke with long swims in Lake Powell…

⌃ Santa Cruz…

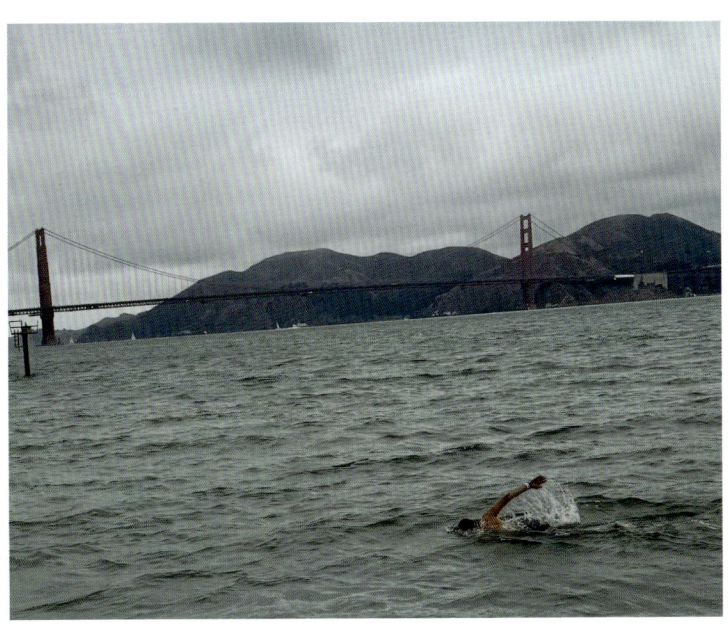

⌃ and San Francisco Bay.

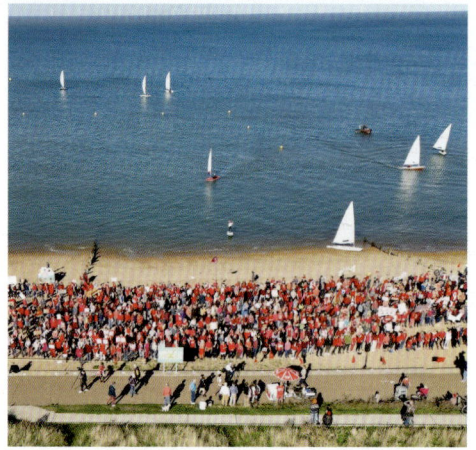

⌃ What do we want? Cleaner water! When do we want it? SOS Whitstable demand Southern Water stop polluting the North Sea in Kent. Credit: @evolutiondrone

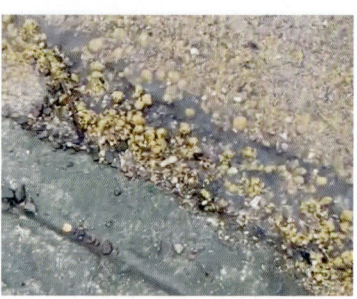

⌃ Actual poo in the Thames. I mean…

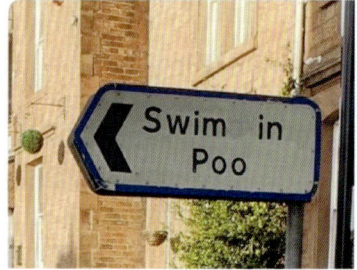

⌃ Quite.

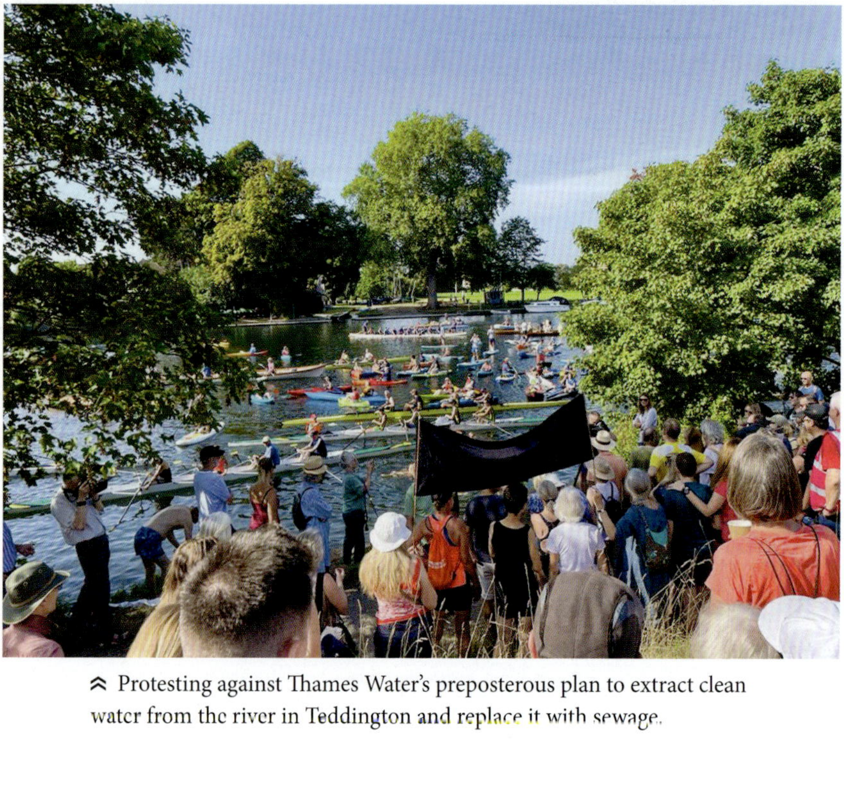

⌃ Protesting against Thames Water's preposterous plan to extract clean water from the river in Teddington and replace it with sewage.

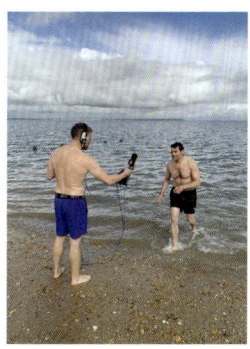

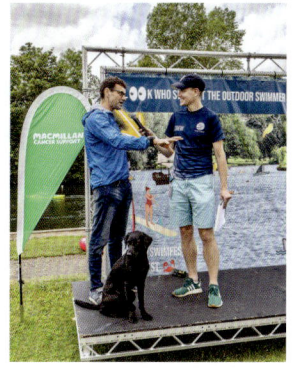

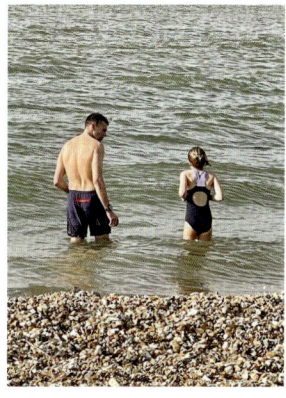

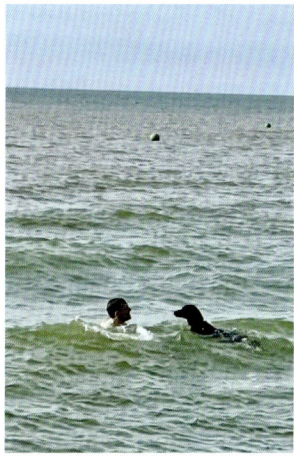

Top Left: I enjoy wild swimming but I don't like to talk about it! With Sam Pinkham on Virgin Radio.

Above: No really, I don't like to talk about it! On stage at the Henley Swim Festival.

Top Right: Persuading a 9-year-old Mary that the North Sea in January is lovely… honestly!

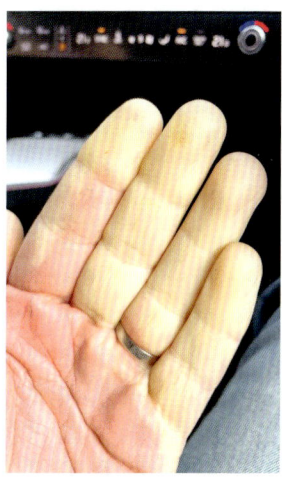

≫ Bella the Labrador thinks of herself as a runner, but she's equally happy joining me for a swim.

≫ Unexpected, somewhat painful, by product of winter swimming!

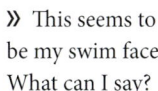

≫ This seems to be my swim face. What can I say?

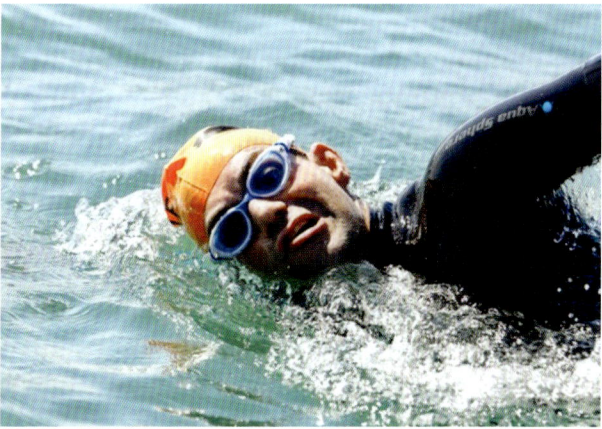

Swimming has the power to change the world. It's been an honour to chat to some of the true greats…

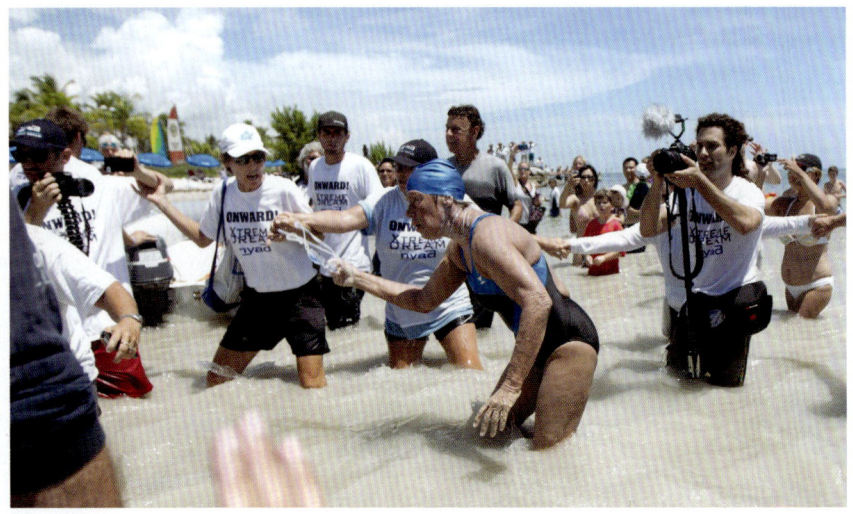

⌃ Diana Nyad inspires millions as she becomes the first person to swim 110 miles from Cuba to Florida without a shark cage – on her fifth attempt, aged 64. © Alamy Images

Right: Gertrude Ederle tears up the rule book of women in sport as she sets off from France to become the first woman to swim the English Channel. Nobody would better her time for decades.
© Getty Images

Bottom left: Lewis Pugh, the first person to swim across the North Pole to highlight the melting of the Arctic Sea ice. © Getty Images

Bottom right: Swimming in the Channel with Channel-swimming legend Sally Minty-Gravett.

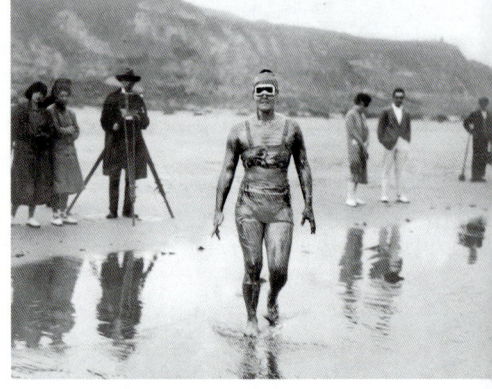

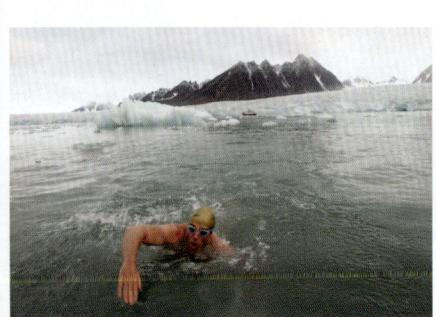

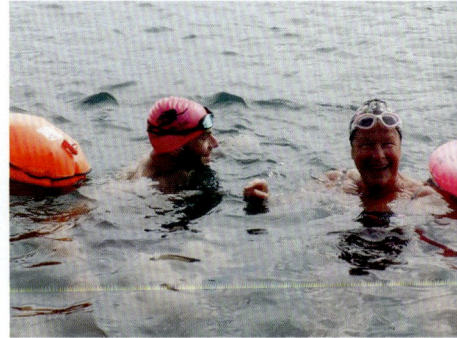

'I started my first winter swim wearing a wetsuit and it took me a year to take the wetsuit off. The ice mile was like this big, deadly, frozen magnet that was pulling me towards it and it was kind of inevitable. But it was an experience like no other.

'I love the fact that I could do a challenge like that, an extreme challenge, in Brockwell Park in London. I wanted to do it on home ground. Brockwell Lido is like my home match, my home stadium, so it just felt right. Very serendipitously, the only other person I know who's done an ice mile there is a lady called Julie. She'd just finished her morning swim and I hadn't seen her in a month or two, and I said, "Oh, I'm just going to... try the ice mile today." And she was like, "Oh, I'll clap you on and cheer you on."

'That really helped. It also made it easier knowing that people were just cracking on with their day and having a coffee, and there wasn't a big fuss or a great hoorah. It took the pressure off in a way and allowed me to focus.

'The hardest part was actually my mind beforehand. I was terrified the night before. I was genuinely lying in bed thinking this is absolutely a stupid idea. I'm going to be that person who's on the news, idiot wild swimmer pushes their luck too far in Brockwell Lido. I was especially scared of the last 200 metres.

'None of my training had gone beyond 1400 metres and it's 1600 for the mile. So those 200 metres felt like a pothole – the further you go into the mile, the narrower it gets, and with each metre you're just getting narrower and narrower and being squeezed tighter and tighter, hoping that at the end of it you come out. I feel horrendous right now, my hands and feet feel like ice cubes, even my lungs feel cold, how the hell am I going to get to 1600 metres? But once I was in the water, I committed to it.

'And actually it flipped once I hit 1400 metres and I suddenly thought, I've only got 200 to go, to do it. So on the day it went from being something I was terrified of to something that was within reach.'

Calum and his brothers have had swimming adventures all over the world. Across Scottish lochs, in Norwegian fjords, across continents in Turkey. Some of these are adventurous bordering on reckless. Once their mother sat Calum down and begged him not to attempt a Scandinavian swim, fearing he could die. He did it anyway:

'It's definitely a balance, yeah. I don't want anyone to encourage themselves to suddenly go and try an ice mile if they're not acclimatised. It's trying to match the recklessness, which can be a positive driving force, with the adventure. I want these experiences. I want a rich life. I want to have those memories of doing something exciting and different. And if I can pair that with relying on experts and expert knowledge, then I know I'm safe.

'There's a great community at the Serpentine. There's a guy called Nick Hungerford who's done three ice miles, and I went for a swim with him and listened to his advice. I got tips on what kind of chocolate was best for your recovery or what kind of tea worked the best. So it's combining the adventurous and the reckless with expert help and advice. That's usually a good Venn diagram sweet spot.'

Speaking of the great community at the Serpentine, it really does exist. It's a camaraderie mixed with a tremendous desire to help one another in all swimming endeavours. As soon as I announced my plan to attempt the Channel, I was inundated with offers of assistance and advice. (The advice being mostly to 'put some weight on, for goodness sake!').

The club has a rich history of producing English Channel swimmers, both solo and relay. A big source of pride for the club is that we were recently inducted into the International Marathon Swimming Hall of Fame. This is proper stuff.

The relevant entry on the IMSHOF website explains that the club was founded in 1864, is based in London's Hyde Park and has a long history of giving back to the swimming community, for instance by raising money for one-to-one swimming lessons for children with physical and sensory disabilities. But, significantly, it notes that the club is a haven for cold water enthusiasts, a major hub for marathon swimmers and has a historic focus on the English Channel, with 82 members having completed solo swims. It then adds:

'Additional marathons completed by members include: Strait of Gibraltar; Lake Geneva/Lac Leman; Lake Zurich; Capri to Naples; Lake Annecy; Round Jersey; Jersey to France; Round Guernsey; Catalina Channel; Manhattan Island; Robben Island; Suez Canal; Cook Strait; plus many crossings of the most famous fresh-water swims in Great Britain such as Loch Lomond; Loch Ness and Lake Windermere.'

That last paragraph reads like a wish list for any aspiring long-distance swimmer. Lake Geneva and Manhattan Island are top of my list, but even in the centre of London you can find an iconic swim marathon.

In the summer, when the Serpentine becomes a lido from 10 a.m., you're only allowed within the buoyed area. Members are allowed almost as far as the Serpentine Bridge, about triple the distance, and to swim the entire length of the lake you need to enter Swim Serpentine, a brilliant event hosted by the organisers of the London Marathon.

Choose between one, two or six laps, each exactly one mile long. I entered in 2022 and loved it. Such a treat to see thousands of people delighting in a lake I'm usually enjoying solo. I chose the two-mile option. It was only afterwards, as I warmed up with a complimentary hot chocolate, that I realised I should have done the full six-mile course. Not just because that would have constituted a proper 'swim marathon', but also, a decade after the London Olympics, because it would have been a replica of the open water swimming course used at the games. It's on my ever-growing to-swim list.

The 1980 Olympic swimming champion Duncan Goodhew is another Serpentine swim club member. He's a relatively recent convert to the pleasures of swimming among the duck poo:

'Well, I kept on walking past the lake with all these crazy people swimming in there and eventually, by 2010, I thought, "I'm going to get an entry form." And I was staggered to see that it was £20 a year. I thought, wow, £20 a year and you get 25% off at the Lido Cafe, so it only takes about four coffees to make your money back. But when I turned it over, there was small print in light grey telling you all the illnesses you could contract from swimming in the Serpentine. So I put it on the shelf and left it.

'And the next year it surfaced again, because I found out that the London 2012 open water swimming was being held in the Serpentine. And I thought, 'God, if they're holding the Olympics there, it must be safe to swim in.'

'And I did a little research and found out they check the water every day. And I thought, "Come on Duncan, you're a soft pool swimmer. You can do this." And so I started with swimming during the summer. The banter is really good down there and you've got a real menagerie of different types of people, and it's very entertaining and lots of ribbing going on. So I was summer only. And everybody kept telling me how great winter swimming was in cold water. But I was like yeah yeah… I just don't get it.

'And eventually, whatever it was, five years later, I thought, "Ah, okay, I'll swim to Christmas." And you get such a buzz out of doing it, it brings you so close to nature and afterwards you get a real, real high. So it's become part of my life. And I do a lot of open water swimming now and I love it.

'I did some research and on average, habitual swimmers are 4% happier than people who don't swim. And if you're an open water swimmer, you're 8% happier. The stats are there to prove it. Open water swimming is extraordinary. You leave all the electronics, you strip off, you go in down to the Serpentine, you get in there and when you get out... If you had to whittle it down to one thing, I'd say you get real contrast in your life. When you have a hot shower afterwards, it's clean, it's hot. And boy, it's one of the best inventions of humankind, especially contrasted to the discomfort of cold water.'

There are two showers next to the Serpentine, both outdoors. The one on the right works better than the one on the left. They're both stone cold, because much as you do crave a lovely, hot shower straight after a freezing swim, it's the last thing you should do. As Duncan knows only too well.

'No hot showers at the Serpentine, thankfully, otherwise you'd get a lot of people emerging from the freezing lake and heading straight into a hot shower. Which is a really ugly thing to do, because you don't recover for the rest of the day. When you've been in cold water for a while and your core temperature has sunk, the capillaries shrink. They contract as you get cold. Your body's trying to get as much heat into its core as possible. So if you go and get hot after being cold for a long period of time, the capillaries open and the blood flows to your skin, robbing the efficient heating process your body's going through.'

When you're in the Serpentine, you feel like you're immersed in nature. But you're not, not really. The lake is completely artificial, built on the whim of an 18th-century royal. It was initially fed by two Thames tributaries, then by the River Thames itself, and now the water's pumped into the lake from three boreholes within Hyde Park. They check water quality daily and ban swimming when the blue-green algae[2] bloom every summer.

It's a similar story in North London. The Hampstead Ponds were originally dug in the 17th and 18th centuries as reservoirs to meet London's growing water demand. Nowadays they're famous for swimming. The men's, women's and mixed ponds – and the eclectic bunch who swim in them – all feature in the 2018 documentary *The Ponds*.

Long before the cameras arrived, the poet Al Alvarez wrote beautifully about his daily dip in the men's pond. It's all about nature: 'Spring is back again, but pale, tentative, washed out, as though after a binge. The Canada geese ignore each other like some ill-matched married couple.' Every entry in his brilliant *Pondlife: A Swimmer's Journal* includes the water temperature (like I say, we do become a little obsessed) and

---

[2]Blue-green algae are not algae but a type of bacteria (called cyanobacteria) that are present in our lakes and rivers. They are very small and can't be seen with the naked eye. When environmental conditions are just right (they like warm, still water with plenty of nutrients), they can multiply quickly forming a 'bloom'.

Blooms appear as a discolouration of the water (often a pea green colour) or as visible scum layers or floating mats. There are no quick or easy remedies for the control of blooms once they appear in a lake or pond.

According to the NHS, blue-green algae may produce several different toxins which are harmful and can cause: skin rashes, nausea, vomiting, stomach pains, fever, headaches and occasionally more serious illness, such as liver and brain damage. Best to give the lakes a wide berth until levels are safe.

how far he manages to swim. Alvarez delights in his swims while simultaneously railing against his advancing years and diminishing physical capabilities. When he's hospitalised after a stroke, fellow swimmers visit with a jar of pond water as a gift. Still got 'pond cred', as he calls it. 'Swimming is good for the soul... and cheaper than therapy.'

The *Times* newspaper columnist Caitlin Moran also swims in Hampstead, in all weathers, but insists she doesn't do it because it's fashionable or she's seeking 'wellness'. She does it because when she emerges from a freezing lake after 10 minutes of agonised breaststroke...

> 'It makes you high as all balls... Do not think you are looking upon a pond of Paltrows when you see cold water swimmers. What you are really looking at is a bunch of hardcore drug bins off their lady-knackers on endorphins. Who needs drugs when I can get off my face cold water swimming?'

And quite frankly Caitlin, so say all of us.

14

Swimming London

Leafy Hampstead, Saturday morning, 6.30 a.m. I'm in a posh cafe sipping an overpriced cappuccino. Normally I feel slightly intimidated whenever I'm in North London, but today I'm feeling like I belong. Not only have I spent £6 on a coffee, I'm also reading a short story by the American author John Cheever. Peak Hampstead.

'The day was beautiful and it seemed to him that a long swim might enlarge and celebrate its beauty.'

Inspired by Cheever's short story 'The Swimmer' and the later film starring Burt Lancaster, my plan for the morning is to swim the length of London. The protagonist in the story is enjoying a lazy day by the pool at a neighbour's house when he realises he can envisage a mental map of all the garden swimming pools forming a kind of river back to his own house. He names the river Lucinda, after his wife, and sets out to travel the length of it.

I'm here for the London version of 'The Swimmer'. Imagine a map of London from north to south as a series of outdoor swimming venues. Essentially, it's a swim down the length of London. Meet at Hampstead Tube, run to Hampstead Ponds for a dip and then to Parliament Hill Lido. Next it's the Serpentine in Hyde Park and on to Brockwell Lido for a final swim and some celebratory pizza. I'm miraculously early, hence the time to read the short story which prompted the morning's exertions.

The story, which begins with such optimism and promise, does take a bit of a turn, though. Pools become colder and harder to swim in, neighbours less welcoming, a storm erupts. As a critic at the time noted, the story turns into 'a quietly devastating journey into one man's heart of darkness'. I like the sound of that somewhat less.

People are starting to gather across the street next to a Transit van and I wander over. The atmosphere is simultaneously jovial and oddball. What did I honestly expect from 50 people who've chosen to begin their weekend swimming down London in the depths of winter? It's a cold February day, but no sign of the rain that's been a staple of the past fortnight.

'That's because Graham's here,' says the organiser. Graham is a local vicar and a regular at The Swimmer. Legend has it that it's never once rained when Graham has turned up. Graham rolls his eyes at the insinuation he has a direct line to whoever controls the weather.

Will Watt has been putting on these monthly swim-run jollies for almost a decade. They're inspired by both Cheever and his own legendary local pool:

'A few years ago, Tooting Lido started something called the London Lido Crawl, where they would start at Tooting and then ride bikes or drive cars up to the Serpentine and then go up to the Ponds in Hampstead. And I did it one year on the bike and then I remember coming back thinking, "I bet you could run this." And so with a friend, Jonathan, who was Tooting club captain at the time, we gave it a go.

'We plotted the route through London's finest parks and ponds – through Hampstead Heath, over Primrose Hill, down through Regent's Park and Hyde Park to the Serpentine. It's a bit more of a slog, but you run through Sloane Square and over Battersea Bridge to get to either Tooting or Brockwell, where we finish now. And so we did it and it was just such a lovely route, and we thought people will like this.'

People did like it. People still do. It soon grew via word of mouth and then an article in the *Guardian*. And so it carried on, a maximum of 50 people meeting early on a Saturday morning to swim the length of London together – once a month and only in winter (the ponds and pools are too busy in summer). At one stage people started turning up in wetsuits using The Swimmer as training for competitive swim-run events like ÖTILLÖ[1], but they soon realised they were at the wrong place. The Swimmer's genius is that it's non-competitive.

The safety briefing essentially consists of, 'Be careful crossing the roads – pretend you're on your own before you cross and don't just follow the herd.' Which is good advice I've since passed on to my kids. And then we're away, jogging and chatting through the undulating, pre-dawn streets of beautiful Hampstead and onto the Heath. Our conversation is straight out of Cheever's short story.

"I drank too much," said Donald Westerhazy, at the edge of the Westerhazys' pool.

"We all drank too much," said Lucinda Merrill.

"It must have been the wine," said Helen Westerhazy. "I drank too much of that claret."

---

[1]ÖTILLÖ, the Swimrun World Championship is, according to the organisers, 'the mother of all swim runs and the origin of the sport… one of the most prestigious endurance races in the world.' Essentially, you run in your wetsuit and swim in your trainers. It's a race between and over 24 islands in a Swedish archipelago. The total distance is 70 kilometres, of which 9 kilometres are open water swimming and 61 are trail running. ÖTILLÖ now lay on swim-run races all over the world. By the time you read this, I'll have completed the one in the Engadin Valley in Switzerland, running on trails through forests of pine trees and swimming in mountain lakes. Can't wait!

It only takes around 20 minutes for those of us who have hangovers to clear them and for us all to arrive at the first swim location, those legendary Hampstead Ponds. These are split by gender, so the women jog on while the rest of us file through the turnstile and into the covered, outdoor changing area. Graham's in high spirits, it's his 60th birthday and he's just used the London Underground for free for the first time with his new senior Oyster Card. He celebrates by launching into a yogic headstand on the cold concrete floor. I can't resist showing off so join him. Soon others go upside down. It's that sort of morning.

Neddy, the protagonist in the Cheever story, is contemptuous of people who don't hurl themselves into swimming pools. There's certainly a bit of that in Hampstead. There's even a diving board. Many of our party hurl themselves off it with abandon. I just can't. It's the ladder for me. I lower myself into the water until I'm waist-deep then let go. It's the only way I'm able to do it. I couldn't tell you why. I have big respect for the divers.

Once in the water, all hangovers really are long forgotten and any residual sleepiness similarly vanishes. Cold water will do that. Some people, myself included, set off on the traditional anti-clockwise lap of the pond, while others are happy to stay near the pontoon and swim and chat. Nobody seems to mind either way. Nobody's hurrying you and nobody's judging how far you've swam or how long you've stayed in the water. You simply get out when you feel like it.

In my rucksack I've brought four pairs of running shorts, which have long since doubled as underwear for me and lately as swimming shorts. The plan is to change into a dry pair after every swim. Except the run from the Ponds to Parliament Hill Lido is very short, only around a mile, so many of us decide to do it wet.

There is lots of banter among the group and a warm welcome from the Hampstead regulars. We grab our bags, start running again and soon arrive at the Lido. I know the hills around here from the annual cross-country race, but before today had no idea there was a 60-metre outdoor pool in the middle of them. Imposing stairs lead to a squat 1930s building housing the changing rooms. Behind the Grade II-listed bricks lies the stainless steel-lined pool. Half of it is almost too shallow to swim.

Some do a dozen or more laps, others just one or two, before heading back to what feels like very luxurious changing facilities. Individual cubicles – and hot showers! The Swimmer veterans sagely advise the rest of us to steer well clear of hot showers after prolonged exposure to cold water. They're right of course.

The thing is to warm up gradually or you increase the risk of something called 'after-drop' – when you feel fine immediately afterwards, but then can start to get colder, start shivering, even grow faint. A few of us decide to ignore the advice due to the fact we're about to run five miles to Hyde Park and reckon the after-drop risk must be fairly low. We sneak into the warm showers, a cubicle per person, and close the curtains. A little slice of illicit heaven!

Will is waiting for us with his transit van in the car park. He offers cakes, bananas, biscuits and backpack transport to the next port of call. Everyone is buzzing. Friendships are being formed. We cheerfully lob our bags into the van and set off towards the Serpentine.

First stop, the top of Primrose Hill for a joyful group photo with London as a backdrop. It feels like the rest of the city is just waking up as we gallop on southwards through Regent's Park and past the Sherlock Holmes Museum at 221B Baker Street. We skirt around the side of Marble Arch into Hyde Park and soon we arrive at the Serpentine car park, which serves both the eponymous art galleries and lake.

We change on what's colloquially known as the beach, aka the wide concrete path on the Serp's southern shore. Lots of proper swimming here, lengths of the buoyed-off swimming area, and lots of messing about too. I join someone in a few metres of splashy butterfly.

When we're all dry(ish) and dressed, we reconvene by the van for the traditional song and dance: strange Europop song by Handsome Dancer called 'Coincidance'. The dance is a ludicrous shoulder shimmy above a wide-legged stance. Everyone joins in. Many know the song from previous editions of The Swimmer and sing along. Still very jovial. And still decidedly oddball.

After the weirdest (and only) car park karaoke of my life, we split into three groups for the longest run of the day, about 7 miles down to Brockwell Lido in Brixton. I tag along with the 'fast' group, but it's not actually that fast and once again there's no competitiveness. Because of the swimming breaks and the zhuzh of cold water, my legs feel all fresh and bouncy, even though they've already run seven miles to get here.

Out of Hyde Park in Knightsbridge, past Harrods and the expensive boutiques on Sloane Street, then through Sloane Square towards Battersea Bridge and, briefly, into Battersea Park. It must be around 10.30 a.m. by now and there are eight of us in the so-called 'fast' group, five men and three women, chatting happily as we run.

There's a half marathon happening in the park. Runners and swim-runners exchange waves and mutual encouragement before we exit and start the climb towards Clapham. We pass the flat my wife and her best friend rented when they first moved to London, which causes me to reminisce at length to my new friends.

From Clapham Common it's downhill all the way to Brixton. When we enter Brockwell Park there's about half a mile left to run. For the first time the pace begins to increase as the more competitive members of our group start stretching their legs. I don't think of myself as competitive – even though all members of my family insist they've never met anyone more so. I see others speed up and remind myself what a glorious morning it's been without any form of competition. I decide to hold back. No racing for me today. After all, as I remind myself, my family are wrong and actually I'm not a competitive person.

And then suddenly I'm sprinting. Turns out I just can't help it. Three minutes later I'm one of three muppets who arrive panting, drained, exhausted at the lido. There's always a few. Will is waiting with the van and a knowing smile:

'One of the first things we agreed is that it should never be competitive. I mean, it's quite a long run, about half a marathon, but we were sort of like, "Come along!" We made it fun, so we would stop and have cake and brandy. A lot of what was going on at the time was triathlons and it was all getting a bit serious, and we were the antidote to that.

'The motto was enjoyment, not endurance. And I mean, anybody who's willing to get up on a Saturday morning at 6 a.m. and run through London and swim through ponds in the winter is going to be an interesting character – just an amazing bunch of people, who are obviously quite committed to life because they'll get up and do that.

'And cold swimming's always got that vibe, but you mix it with running and experiencing London in a completely different way. It is a bit of alchemy. There's a unique euphoria on people's faces when they finish.'

Or, in my case, having inadvertently sprinted the final half mile, the expression is a mixture of sheepish and exhausted. I collect my rucksack from the van and head for the final swim of the morning.

Brockwell Lido is another London gem. A 50-metre unheated outdoor pool opened in 1937 and closed for good in 1990. It reopened in 1994 thanks to a committed local campaign to save it. Two ex-council employees took on the running of the pool for the community. The lido remains a beacon to that spirit, as well as serving amazing pizza.

It's a funny thing, but despite running around 14 miles and swimming four times in freezing water, nobody is tired. We all feel like we can springboard into the rest of the weekend. After a ton of pizza, of course. When everyone has arrived in Brixton and finished swimming, a huge pile of steaming flat boxes emerges from the cafe. You've never seen food disappear as quickly as those pizzas. We may not be fatigued, but we are famished.

Everybody has had an adventure. Everybody has made new friends. Phone numbers are exchanged. That first time, when I chat to Will over pizza, I'm horrified to discover that The Swimmer's days in London may be numbered, but then apparently that's what he always says:

'Every year I say I'm never doing it next year, it's too much like hard work, and then I always do because you see so many smiling faces at the end, and you can go for a pint with them and everyone's really funny, and having a laugh is a lovely, lovely thing just to be part of, never mind having created it.'

Will has since created a version of The Swimmer in Copenhagen (alongside the brilliantly named Copen Water Swimmers), as well as devising non-competitive swim-run adventures all over the UK. He's invented the RuckRaft, a fully inflatable raft that comes with a giant dry bag and backpack handles, which can be easily carried over land and towed through water. I can't wait to join one of his cross-country swim-runs in Devon, Snowdonia or the Lake District.

I have a huge grin on my face as I leave Brixton to head home. As Will tells everyone who completes The Swimmer: 'You've done more in a morning than most people manage in a month.'

15

Swimming Ice

I never intended to buy an ice bath. I don't remember ever making a conscious decision to part with some money in exchange for one. Buying an ice bath is something that sort of just happened to me.

It was mid-April, so the Serpentine was beginning to warm up and the dawn swim was changing. I do love those spring mornings: being in the water as the first hint of daylight appears above the city of London. Some mornings you can see the sun rising over one side of the lake and turn around to see the moon setting over the other. You can also spend much longer in the water, so your winter 10-minute dip morphs into a proper half hour, mile-long swim.

The light, the fact it's so much easier to get into water that's fresh not freezing and the appearance of a few more early swimmers – all surefire signs that spring has sprung. Which, of course, means summer's on its way, all great, all exciting. But it also means the water won't be cold again for at least seven months. And I know from previous years how much I'll miss that.

The water temperature occupies an unhealthy amount of a Serpentine swimmer's thoughts. The exact number – complete to the nearest decimal point – is sent out on the Serp's X account every day. And I do mean every day. They take this very seriously. They have three digital thermometers and tweet the average temperature between them, just to make sure it's bang on. The general feeling among those of us who love the cold is: single figures is proper, below five is ideal. Above 15 is lovely, but…

On the way home from work that fateful day, my Brompton picked up a puncture and I ended up on the train. I found myself in an empty carriage. I took a seat and pulled out my phone as the train pulled out of the station. Everything seemed to happen very quickly after that.

The journey from London Waterloo to Barnes takes 22 minutes. In those 22 minutes, I somehow managed to do all of the following: google ice baths, click on the first likely link (theicebath.co), browse the products on offer, like the look of their oval ice bath, come up with several questions, text the contact number, receive a call from a likeable man called Luke who owns the company, have my questions answered ('It's fine to keep the ice bath permanently at 2 degrees and it costs around 20p a day in electricity'), find out about how and why he started the company, discover he's also a competitive bodybuilder, tell him I'll call him back if I decide to place an order, call him straight back and place an order. I finish paying just as the train slows down at Barnes Station.

I was ridiculously pleased as I barrelled through the front door. 'Hey, Caroline, guess what just happened?!' Caroline immediately – and correctly – diagnoses a middle-class male midlife crisis. Most of my friends and family agree. How do you know if somebody gets into cold water? They will tell you.

I've got to say, though, much as I made the purchase on a whim, I was right to buy the ice bath. I mean I absolutely hate it obviously; it makes me hurt. But I also adore it and climb in every day; it makes me feel wonderful.

People often ask me how to mitigate the dark places I must find myself in during a 100-mile run or an eight-hour swim.

They're asking the wrong question. It's not dark. You peel back the layers and what you find underneath is just love and light. And that's the case for all of us. Under all the crap that life chucks on top of us, under childhood trauma and losing your keys this morning and that BMW driver cutting you up just now, I believe we're all infinitesimal shards of the same universal force and it's a force for good.

At mile 25 of the 2023 London Marathon, I saw our eight-year-old daughter Mary at the side of the road. It was hot inside the massive minion costume I was running in and I was close to my physical limit. She was holding a sign saying, 'You're one in a minion daddy!' I stopped to give Mary a hug and a kiss before carrying on along the Embankment. The whole episode took around 10 seconds.

I was in floods of tears as I ran towards Westminster Bridge and the finish, and, according to Caroline, so was Mary. Tears of joy, verging on rapture. The layers were peeled back to pure love. And Mary, being eight, obviously had fewer layers to peel back. Though perhaps it was also the fact she'd been given a sweaty kiss through the eye hole of a giant minion!

So believe me, it's not a dark place. But that's not to say it doesn't hurt. The German cyclist Jens Voigt famously has the phrase 'Shut up legs' tattooed on his thighs. The pain is the point. Which brings us back to the ice bath.

My morning regime goes like this. The first alarm is a vibration on my watch, so as not to wake Caroline. It frequently fails to wake me either, so two minutes later an old iPhone tinkles with its 'first light' alarm tone. I can't recommend rousing yourself from your dreams with a gently increasing mellow tune highly enough. My old alarm would wrench me from sleep with a hefty dose of fight or flight. This is a soft launch into the day.

I try to remember to smile and think positive, happy thoughts first thing. As if training my brain for the day ahead.

Well begun is half done, as my gran used to say. I also offer up some gratitude and a quiet prayer. If all goes to plan, I can feel positive energy coursing through me as I swing my legs on to the floor. Which is when Mike Tyson punches me in the solar plexus. The ice bath. My appointment with the least comfortable seat in South West London.

'Remember how good you'll feel afterwards,' I say to myself as I grab the towel that lives on the sitting room door and head for the garden like I'm approaching the gallows. I still can't believe I'm going to go through with this. 'Remember how good you'll feel,' I repeat as I slide open the back door trying not to wake the dog. 'Remember how good,' I say as I take the lid off the ice bath and lean it against the house. It's too late now. Somehow the act of removing the lid also removes any doubt about what's about to happen. I climb the stairs, and swing my legs over the edge and into the water. I question my life choices as the cold bites into my lower half.

And then, with a long exhale, I look up to the sky and submerge up to my shoulders, hands clenched on thighs. Let the torture begin: two minutes minimum, five max. Sometimes I'll literally count the seconds, inhale for five, exhale for 10 – eight times is two minutes. It actually gets easier after a minute or so, and there's a kind of sweet spot between the initial horror and the later pain in your extremities. I'll also dunk my head forwards into the water before getting out, but compared to the first freezing shock or the pain in my hands and feet, that bit is quite easy.

It's a similar start to the day whenever I'm commuting from Whitstable. You've got to be lucky (or unlucky) with the tides to get a swim in before driving to work. One January morning I was lucky (unlucky) and high tide was perfectly timed at 4 a.m. I arrived on the beach in the pitch dark, no lights on the seafront. I stood on the stones wearing nothing but shorts and goggles. The wind coming off the sea was not quite fierce enough to allow me to abandon this entire escapade and head for the warmth of the car and clothes.

Reach the water and the trick is to keep walking as the icy water laps around your ankles, shins, knees, thighs... When it's up to your hips, fall forwards into its spiky embrace. It's not as bad as all that, you tell yourself, as you acclimatise with a stroke or two of breaststroke. Then don't stop to think, simply plunge your face into the waves and start a steady front crawl. The face hurts for longest. Breathe every three strokes, a momentary respite every time. Within a dozen breaths you realise it's as good as it's going to get, just keep swimming for as long as you can bear. Two minutes... three... five... Keep checking you're not being dragged too deep by the current... eight minutes... hands and feet hurting now... 10 minutes... 11... Remind yourself that the Channel crossing will be warmer than this... 12... Finally back to the shore, numb, shivering, utterly exhilarated. And dry, dress and drive to work.

Ice bath dip and North Sea swim – both versions of the granny rule: 'Eat your carrots before pudding.' When the first thing you do is swap the blissful comfort of the duvet for the sharp bite of freezing water (eating your carrots), the rest of your day feels like an apple pie.

There are medical benefits too. Recent research into the effects of freezing water has revealed how it can help with injury recovery, reduce inflammation, and enhance overall physical and mental well-being.

After intense physical activity, microscopic tears occur in muscle fibres, leading to inflammation and the characteristic muscle pain known as delayed onset muscle soreness (DOMS). Cold water helps constrict blood vessels and reduce metabolic activity, which in turn limits the buildup of waste products like lactic acid that cause the soreness. When the body warms back up after the bath, blood flow increases, flushing out the waste products, and bringing in fresh oxygen and nutrients to repair the damaged tissues. This process accelerates recovery, allowing athletes to get back to training sooner.

Cold exposure is a well-documented method for reducing inflammation all over the body, which has been linked to chronic illnesses and autoimmune conditions. By lowering the temperature of muscle tissues, ice baths help to reduce swelling and numb pain. The cold causes blood vessels to constrict, limiting the amount of inflammatory fluid that accumulates in the tissues and preventing further damage. This can be particularly helpful for people recovering from injuries or surgeries.

Although it may seem counterintuitive, ice baths actually improve circulation over time. The blood vessels constrict but once the body warms up, they dilate, which increases circulation.

Cold exposure has also been linked to a significant boost in immune function. Regular ice baths trigger a stress response in the body, which activates the immune system. This process increases the production of white blood cells, which are essential for fighting off infections.

In terms of mental health benefits, immersion in cold water triggers the release of endorphins, the body's natural mood enhancers. This can result in a sense of euphoria and relief from stress or anxiety. Furthermore, the mental discipline required to endure the discomfort of an ice bath also has psychological benefits, promoting resilience and enhancing the ability to manage stress. The contrast between the shock of the cold and the feeling of invigoration afterwards can provide a mental 'reset'.

Some studies suggest that cold water immersion can improve sleep quality. The drop in body temperature triggers a natural cooling effect, which signals the body that it's time to rest. As the body warms back up afterwards, it induces a relaxation response that can make falling asleep easier.

I'm not sure about that last one, though. I once (and only once) made the mistake of heading for the ice bath after reading Mary her bedtime story. I felt wonderful straight afterwards, of course, but an hour later remember lying in bed trying to sleep, feeling like I'd necked three espresso martinis.

As to the point about the cold giving you a mental reset – that one definitely works. One of the most dramatic mood changes I've ever experienced came one freezing Sunday evening in the North Sea. It literally turned my frown upside down – and did so in seconds. In the freezing water, you don't think, you're just there. It's like you're being cleansed of frustrations. Cold temperatures also stimulate the vagus nerve, which is the longest nerve in the body and acts as a counterbalance to our fight or flight system.

And there's definitely something to be said for 'feeling' the seasons, a step up from eating seasonally. We're lucky to live in heated homes and travel in heated cars. For the short periods of time we're outside in winter, we make sure to 'wrap up warm'. How do our bodies even know it's winter?

And finally, it's an amazing fact that cold water exposure actually slows down the ageing process. There's proper science to prove it. It's all about your telomeres. These are the protective coverings at the end of chromosomes that shorten with each cell division. Cold water promotes longer telomeres, protecting your DNA. It also increases levels of RBM3 and RTN3, which are protective proteins that help prevent brain degeneration. And there's even evidence to show that ice baths reduce the appearance of wrinkles and fine lines on skin.

But more than any of that, cold water quite simply 'feels' right – life-giving and life-affirming. You don't have to buy an ice bath – just start with a cold shower. It's nowhere near as cold, but it's still great. Start with your usual warm shower and do what you do. Before you get out, turn the temperature control to fully cold. There's usually a lag, which helps. And when the cold water begins, simply stay under it for as long as you can. Even 10 seconds will give you a boost. Build it up slowly. Once you're up to two minutes, you've basically won.

Caroline, who was initially dubious about that spontaneous ice bath purchase on the train to Barnes now gets in at least once a week. Friends come round and sometimes, after a glass of wine or two, decide to give it a try. Nobody regrets it. Even our youngest daughter Mary will get into the ice bath, if only very briefly, then sprint round the garden like a loony. Cold water immersion is objectively horrific, but who doesn't want to feel like sprinting round the garden like a loony?

16

Swimming Downhill V

Once I start understanding the stroke, the whole process seems to speed up. As, obviously, does my swimming. Soon Ray has me buying something called a 'centre line snorkel' which looks like a cross between something you take on your summer holidays and something from a bondage dungeon. It helps you do your drills without having to think about breathing. It also makes you look decidedly odd as you splash up and down lane three of the 20-metre gym pool under a skyscraper in the city of London.

I have a secret game I like to play. I note the occasional snide glances I receive as I do my drills: kicking behind a tow float or swimming with one arm and a paddle (the 'advanced single arm paddle' drill) or some other such contrivance designed to get the correct motion into my muscle memory. I'm concentrating on executing correctly, but generally travelling at a snail's pace. I'm aware I look idiotic and frequently fellow swimmers will subtly let me know just how idiotic. Just with a glance at the turn or a smirk as they swim past.

But after 20 minutes or so of drills I'm allowed off the leash to swim properly for the next 20. That's when I enjoy myself. That's when I start doing the overtaking. Even underwater, I suspect it's pretty obvious to everyone how pleased with myself I am. This is what the drills were for, everyone.

By now swimming feels genuinely easy. I frequently find myself doing tumble turns and marvelling at how quickly the last 20 metres went by. I used to dread those tumble turns, knowing I'd be out of breath at the end of them. Now, suddenly, miraculously, I look forward to them with no shortness of breath whatsoever. Like I say, everything feels easy. Confidence grows and grows.

Finally, just before Ray gleefully takes a much-deserved month off to spend April house-sitting for a triathlete friend in the Caribbean, he tells me to relax my arms when they're out of the water. He calls it 'noodle arms'. Pretend your arms are overcooked spaghetti and you're throwing them far in front of you. Never mind the splash. I do so, and instantly feel quicker and stronger.

He shows me a recording of me from above and tells me I've begun to look like a proper open water swimmer. And he's right, I do. The stroke bears little resemblance to the shoulder-driven nonsense I arrived with five months ago. I begin to believe in my swimming. On a good day, I even believe in my solo Channel attempt. I might just do this... If only people would stop telling me to put on weight.

A case in point is the actor Will Ellis. Apart from being a big star – as a nasty piece of work – in *Eastenders*, he's a kind and gentle man, pretty much an elite swimmer and one of Ray's star pupils, as well as being coached by Sally Minty-Gravett. I had called him out of the blue one afternoon having never met him, and he couldn't have been more helpful and giving. He was planning his own solo assault on the Channel and he stayed on the phone with me for over an hour, offering advice and expertise. We kept in touch on WhatsApp:

'It sounds like you need to really think about gaining a few pounds now as you'll struggle to do so in the spring when cold-water swimming in earnest. Let me know if I can help: but essentially it's eating a healthy amount and supplementing with post-workout protein shakes and lots of liquids (feeds) when swimming. FWIW there are some pilots (not yours) who simply won't take a swimmer if they appear lean on the day…

'Aaaaand one more thing – you should visit us here in Brighton for a swim at the Sea Lanes while winter is still here – 50m pool, 18 degrees… so chilly-ish by conventional swimming pool standards. Have a long swim in that now as a marker. Catch up soon! W

'PS I spent a fortune on a swim-specific nutritionist last year and I'm delighted to share all the information…'

See what I mean about the swimming community? So helpful – and just a tiny bit naggy! Sally also keeps telling me to put on some weight. As does Ray. As does every Serpentine Swim Club member with Channel 'previous' when they find out I'm hoping to swim to France.

And the truth is I do try, but my heart isn't in it. I love every aspect of open water swimming – except the need for a layer of fat for both insulation and buoyancy. And even if my heart was in it, I'd struggle to put on the necessary ballast. Not with a weekly training regime that looks like this:

Running: four or five times a week. Running this much is frowned upon in the ultra-swimming community as it burns too many calories and keeps you too lean. But the fact is, I'm chair of my local running club, Barnes Runners, so can hardly give it up entirely. And, second, I love – and need – my runs. So there.

Weight training: three times-a-week. I've adapted this to make it more swim-specific and it's very necessary for people over 40 (for everyone actually) to prevent muscle atrophy and keep the bones healthy. Since I've started throwing metal around in the gym, my running has got slower, but I've never felt fitter.

Cycle commutes: about 40 minutes each way every weekday morning on my trusty Brompton. Love this too. Especially as on the way to work I stop halfway at…

The Serpentine: the big lake in the middle of Hyde Park. In the summer it's light and gorgeous, and you can have a proper swim of up to a mile and it makes you feel like you're on holiday. And in winter it's cold and dark, and often you're the only one there and the icy waters give you a huge boost. That and duck poo, which is everywhere.

Swimming: every chance I can get. I've joined gyms all over London so I'm never too far from a lane. During the winter I've been doing Ray's drills four or five times a week. And as the blossom has started to appear on the trees and my swimming stroke has become more secure, my weekly mileage has gradually increased. During peak training, I manage two 25-mile-swim weeks. And yes, I now know what 'swimming downhill' feels like. It's ace.

My final lesson with Ray ends with my goggles suffering a total fail five minutes before the end. The suction on the left eye comes loose and water pours in whenever I put my head underwater. This is the first time I've 'swum through' a pair of goggles and it feels significant. I swim on with closed eyes, discarded goggles and a big smile. Ray is filming from above and telling me what to do for homework. When we finish, I stand a little taller in the water as if I've come through another aquatic rite of passage.

Looking at the footage later, I notice I was swimming diagonally across the pool, which Ray was too polite to mention. It looks faintly ridiculous. But even now I find myself searching up that file from time to time and watching myself swimming into the corner. It was the first day I began to feel like 'a swimmer'.

17

Swimming Hours

One of the many things I love about the world of outdoor swimming is that swims tend to be measured in time rather than distance. It seems a far less egocentric metric; more accepting of things as they are.

Michael Singer, the American spiritualist and author of the multi-million bestselling *The Untethered Soul*, will tell you that under no circumstances should the universe in front of you be the way you want it to be. It should simply be the way that it is. And if you try and bend the universe to your will – force it to be the way you want – then you're not going to mess up the universe. You're going to mess up yourself.

That's how training for something like a Channel swim feels. You can't affect the tides, the swell, the water temperature. You don't worry too much about how far or fast you're swimming. You set yourself a time target and quietly accept everything else as it presents itself on the day. Even the official Channel qualifying swim is 'six hours in water colder than 16 degrees'. There's no mention of how far you have to swim in that time.

I've heard people insist that there's a kind of tacit macho rule among outdoor swimmers that makes fear of the cold a subject they don't discuss. In my experience, it's quite the opposite. Fear of the cold is the ONLY subject. And we respect and celebrate everyone who conquers that fear. Which in fact we all do every single time we enter the water. Every swim is a tiny act of bravery. Even in summer and especially in winter.

David Walliams famously swam the Channel for Sport Relief. On the day a camera crew followed his every movement and his progress was documented to millions every few minutes on Radio 1. What nobody saw or heard about were the hours of hard training he endured in the year leading up to the swim. He was on tour around the UK at the time and in every city he'd head to the nearest bit of coast or open water and, literally, put the hours in, slowly building up his endurance and ability to withstand the cold.

I caught up with David one morning on the show when he was publicising his latest kids' book and I ambushed him with question after question about Channel swimming (for the record the book was *Astrochimp* and it's very funny. Sorry David – and thank you!):

> 'The hardest bit was getting used to the cold, because that makes you miserable. It's just relentless. You know what I mean? It doesn't change. Even if you swim as hard as you can, it's still your core temperature. I once swam in the North Sea in Newcastle in December. I had a wetsuit on, but you get claw hands and claw feet where you can't even cup your hand to swim anymore.'

I tell David I've experienced very similar feelings, also in the North Sea, in Kent, and it turns out we have similar coping strategies:

> 'If you're just going to moan, then it's not going to get you anywhere. So don't moan about the cold because nothing can be done. It's not going to change. But it's the length of time as well, which is unusual. I'd do eight-hour training

swims in Dover Harbour. Get in at 9 a.m., get out at 5 p.m. And without having got out or had any food.

'And you know when people say, "Would you do it again?" No. No! I did it, it wasn't that much fun, but it's a nice achievement. It's nice when it's over. Although oddly I did feel a little bereft when it was over. I'd been working so hard towards it for so long. And suddenly it's like, "Oh, it was a purpose."'

Which is what I'm finding. You need quite a lot of motivation to spend hours on your own swimming in the cold sea. Living as I do in London, the bulk of my long swim training has been in heated pools. There were pre-dawn swims in the Serpentine and Whitstable, too, but they never lasted more than half an hour. I had work to get to. My first long sea swim of the year had happened the weekend before I chatted with David and I wasted little time telling him about how tough it was, but he was sweetly supportive:

'Okay, yeah, it's grim, isn't it? Actually when you get to the day, it's exciting, because when you do an eight-hour training swim, you don't get a round of applause when you finish. So yeah, the day was exciting. It started very early, I think at 4 a.m. You're trying to eat some porridge or something. And I said goodbye to my mum and dad on the beach. And it was live on Radio 1. And, I mean, that was exciting. You feel like you're at the centre of something.

'And when you start, it's a bit nerve wracking, because you've got all this adrenaline. It's that thing like a school cross-country run. You come out of the traps a bit too fast, everyone sprints and you're a kid, you just sprint. So I just had to keep calm.

'I said to Greg, my coach, "Don't tell me until we're halfway." He says, "You're halfway." And I feel like it's one of those things, it's like going up and down a mountain; going up, but once you're at the top, it suddenly feels like you're freewheeling – you know that lovely thing on a bike when you're going down a hill.

'So for some reason, psychologically, the second part felt great and it was really exciting. And then the real thrill was when I got towards France, for the first time in 10 hours I could see the bottom. And when I saw the bottom, it was like, "Yes." And that was a lovely, lovely feeling.'

A 'lovely, lovely feeling' – I've spent over a year trying to imagine and doing everything I can to manifest that feeling.

The week before chatting with David I'd driven my wife and daughters to Heathrow airport and carried on down to the coast. They were off to Stockholm to see Taylor Swift begin the European leg of her billion-dollar world tour, while I was aiming to create my own 'Cruel Summer' in Dorset. There was no 'Bad Blood' as I dropped them at terminal two and pointed the 'Getaway Car' towards Bournemouth to continue my swimming 'Love Story' (I'll stop now).

There's a group called the Durley Swimmers who meet on every weekend morning from May to September just west of Bournemouth Pier. There is always support on the beach for swims up to seven hours. On the longer swims feeds are provided to keep people going. A suggested donation of £3 per swim goes towards costs. The group is run completely by volunteers with the philosophy of swimmers supporting swimmers.

Another suggestion is that for every four swims (two full weekends), swimmers could look to donate one morning by being on the beach and supporting others. A parkrun-like philosophy and it works brilliantly. I emailed the group one June to ask if I could come along and Marcus replied straightaway with a friendly, 'Yes, of course'.

I never made it that June. Life got in the way and I hadn't yet realised how much planning needs to go around swims. It's not like 'grab your shoes and find a spare hour to go for a run.' Swimming needs organisation.

The following May, as my family 'Shake It Off' in Stockholm, I try again. No emails this time, I decide to simply turn up and say hi. It's 10 a.m. when I arrive and I can see four or five swimmers already in the water, their garish tow floats slowly sliding across the bay. The weather is glorious, cotton buds of white clouds scudding across the blue sky on a warm breeze. The sand feels fantastic underfoot.

I start towards the obvious Durley Swimmers' meeting point, but at the last moment lose confidence and turn the other way. For reasons that I can't quite fathom (still), I suddenly decide to get the swim done alone. I've brought a bag to the beach containing: one wetsuit, which I won't wear, one car key which I hope won't be stolen, one swim cap, one pair of new goggles, one plain wholemeal pitta bread and one Kind Dark Chocolate Nuts & Sea Salt snack bar. I'm wearing swim shorts under my jeans. I swiftly remove the trousers and add them to the bag, which will stay on the beach. Grabbing the cap and goggles I wade out into the sea. I'm nervous.

The water is still quite cold. It tends to take much of the summer to warm up and this is still mid-May. I mustn't overthink, just get swimming. Utilising the lessons I've learned in the Whitstable sea and icy Serpentine in winter, I keep moving forwards. I wade into the shallows and as soon as the water reaches waist height, take the plunge and start swimming. In the depths of January I'll typically stay in the water for 10 minutes or so. Today I'm determined to tough it out for four hours. The qualification swim for the Channel stipulates six; four seems a good start. Plus if I manage the full four hours, it'll mean I'll be swimming for longer than I'm driving today – and for some reason that seems important to me.

After 10 tough minutes, I decide that I can downgrade four hours to a more manageable 20 minutes and class that as a successful swim. I can't seem to get warm and my rule of thumb is that 20 minutes constitutes exercise and can be added to my somewhat obsessive daily list of athletic endeavours. It's been years since I wrote 'rest day' on that list.

Water as cool as this feels like a piping hot bath to the greatest ice swimmer alive today, Lewis Pugh. Dubbed the 'Sir Edmund Hillary of swimming', he's the first person to complete a long-distance swim in every ocean of the world and he frequently swims in vulnerable ecosystems to draw attention to their plight.

In 2007, Lewis became the first person to swim across the North Pole. Three years later, he swam across a glacial lake on Mount Everest. And in 2018 he swam the 328-mile *length* of the English Channel. The width is proving tricky enough for me. He lives in Plymouth and is the first United Nations Patron of the Oceans:

'We are in a race against time to save our oceans. We are facing an environmental catastrophe and I cannot describe it in any other way. I'm 54 years old. In my lifetime, we've lost over 70% of the world's wildlife. I mean, think about that: over 70% of the world's wildlife. And every year we face more floods, more droughts, more storms, more wildfires, and they're getting more and more destructive.

'When I did my first swim in the high Arctic, so in the Norwegian Arctic, right up against the Arctic sea ice, the sea temperature was 3 degrees. I went back 12 years later and it had risen to 10 degrees Celsius. So just to reiterate, it had gone from 3 degrees Celsius to 10 degrees Celsius in just 12 years, right up against the Arctic sea ice.

'Every year I just see glaciers retreating. And the reality is that now the glaciers are moving faster than our world leaders, and we pour raw sewage into our rivers and coral reefs are dying. And there are plenty of parts of the world now where you get air temperatures over 50 degrees Celsius. So in summary, what I'm saying is we're facing an environmental catastrophe and we are now in an absolute race against time to save the planet.'

If anything, he's understating the urgency. If it's a race, then the bell has rung for the final lap, the Kenyans have kicked for home and we've somehow got to keep up. As if to reinforce Lewis' point, when I speak to him in May – on coincidentally the afternoon before my Bournemouth swim – the water temperature in Plymouth is around 10 degrees.

If you go for a swim in the high Arctic in July, north of the island of Spitsbergen, right up against the Arctic Sea ice, then the water temperature will be between 10 and 12 degrees Celsius. We're talking 80 degrees north and only a few hundred kilometres to the North Pole. This summer, the water temperature will be the same as it is on the English Riviera in May. And when Lewis started in 2005, that Arctic water was 3 degrees.

Of course many of the greatest scientific minds in the world are working on this, seeking solutions that can change the course we seem to be inexorably steering. I ask Lewis whether he believes there's any cause for optimism:

'Well, certainly in terms of marine protected areas. There's been a lot of progress on that. Obviously there's so much more we can do, but that gives me hope that nations have come together now and have agreed that by 2030 at least 30% of the world's oceans and land will be designated as protected areas. That's a great first step.

'In terms of solar, the price of that is coming down fantastically. There's so much more awareness, especially with the youth, which is very, very heartening. I mean, when

I started this back in the early 2000s, I really did feel like a voice in the wilderness. Now there are lots of people talking about how important it is, but we now need to move beyond words and into hardcore, fast action.'

Lewis was born in Devon and moved to South Africa when he was 10. His parents bought a house on a beach and his high school classroom overlooked the sea. His physical education lessons took place on the sand. It was, as he says, 'perfect'. And when he started swimming, he simply adored it. The sea brought him deep joy. And he's never stopped. Now each year he tries to make his big swims a little harder and more challenging than the year before. He hopes to still be swimming into his 90s.

'It really is the one sport in the world where you can do it much, much later in life. I'm 54 years old. I hope it doesn't sound arrogant to say, but I'm at the top of my game at the moment. If you think about it, I think I'm only halfway through my career, because I want to push right the way through to 90.'

Lewis trains every day of the week for 51 weeks a year. He only takes a week off after a big expedition. Seven days' rest and then back to training. Lots of swimming, of course, and kayaking, running, weights. We have that in common at least – commitment to training. And if I thought I was mentally tough, it's nothing compared to Lewis. He's a real inspiration as I swim miserably along in Bournemouth and guiltily recall our conversation of the previous evening. I'd even asked him what it's like to be an inspiration, how he does it:

'When I dive in, I am 100% committed. There's a difference between motivation and inspiration, though. The only person who can motivate yourself is you. Motivation comes from the inside. Inspiration can come from the outside. You can see somebody do a swim or a run, or somebody work really, really hard at school or university and achieve success in business… and that can inspire you. And you look at your own life and you think to yourself, "Am I giving 100%?"'

It's the question I ask myself as I contemplate cutting this four-hour training swim to 20 minutes. Am I giving 100%? I resolve to swim for an hour in one direction, away from the pier towards Sandbanks, before coming back the same way. At least then I'll have managed two hours, the length of a one-way car journey from home. And just in case, I'm swimming in the shallows: the beach is right there if I truly need to get out.

I start to practise 'radical acceptance'. Suffering doesn't come directly from pain (or cold) but from my attachment to the pain (cold). I stop judging the water temperature, stop obsessing about how miserable it's making me and accept things for what they are. And it really helps.

Every 10 minutes or so my watch vibrates to let me know I've covered 500 metres. I'm aiming for a maximum of 10 minutes per vibration, which equates to a two-minute 100 metres and the speed at which official Channel pilots are apparently pleased to see you swimming. It turns out to be one second over. I don't stress about it and then 30 minutes have gone by, 40, 50… If I turn back now I'll have swum for an hour and 40, which is a decent effort for a first crack at a long, cold swim. But I don't turn back. I keep going until the sixth vibration and swim a large arc before heading back towards Bournemouth beach.

The current is with me on the way back so my speed improves, as does my mood. A few minutes short of two hours and I'm scrambling back on to the sand in search of the pitta. It's all I've been thinking about for the past 40 minutes. That, and the fact I can probably manage the full four hours.

The sight of my feet shocks me as I emerge on to the sand. I would describe myself as ethnically 'white', although of course I'm not actually white, I'm a sort of pinkish beige. After two hours' swimming, my feet have become pristine white. The colour of a Transit van as it rolls off the production line. They're also tricky to balance on. This is... interesting.

The pitta takes all of 15 seconds to scoff and I'm straight back into the sea on those weird unsteady feet of mine. Same again and I'm done. Easy, I think. Continue with the whole radical acceptance thing and crack on.

The next hour might well be the hardest mental and physical test I've ever endured. Just 20 minutes in, barely over halfway overall and I'm really struggling. The scale of what's still to come, ANOTHER HOUR AND 40 MINUTES, terrifies me. The beach is JUST THERE. The temptation to give up and find a way to call this a win is overwhelming. Good job Lewis Pugh's interview is still so fresh in my mind:

'You've got to dig into the reason why you're doing these things. Right? So for me, when I was preparing to swim across the North Pole, I didn't know that I would get to the other end. I mean, I really didn't. The world is divided between pioneers and followers. You are either a pioneer or you're a follower and you can't be both. And I remember standing on the edge looking into the water. The water's completely black, completely black. And I had this dreadful thought as I was just about to go into the water, thinking to myself, "Gosh, if things go horribly wrong now, how long will it take for my frozen corpse to sink all the way to the bottom of the Arctic Ocean?" A terrible thought to have.

'So just before I'm getting in the water, I do a brain flush. This is really important, just to clean out the brain very, very quickly. And then I do a mental stacking process. I go all the way back to the beginning of my life and I start thinking about all the successful swims I've done, and I just remember each and every one of them. I then go to the end of my life, and I try and visualise what I'm hoping to achieve. And ultimately, it's always about self-belief. And where does self-belief come from? Self-belief comes from different places for different people, but one has to at that moment believe that, for me, what I was doing was really important in terms of trying to protect the Arctic, which I felt so deeply about.

'Purpose will get you in the water, but it won't keep you in freezing cold water, because it's so painful. A lot of people now have done ice miles and it's a little bit of a misnomer that, because sometimes these swims are in 4 degrees Celsius. There's a vast difference between 4 degrees and zero, and again between zero and minus 1.7.

'Water's a fascinating substance. So between zero and 100, and I'm talking about fresh water at sea level, between zero and 100, it's a liquid. Above 100, it changes completely. It becomes a gas. Below zero, it changes from a liquid into a solid. So there's a certain tipping point at which everything changes. Now, there is a vast, vast, vast difference between swimming in zero and minus 1.7. The pain is absolutely astronomical and, when you enter that water, the feeling is one of a death zone. So even though purpose may be able to get you in that water, you have to be super-sharp, super-focused to be able to swim in that type of water.

'When the United Nations generously appointed me as the United Nations Patron of the Oceans, they said, "Lewis, you have one job. And that's to be a voice for the world's oceans and all the magnificent wildlife that live in our oceans." That's a task that I try to undertake every single day. And I use swimming to try and shine a light on those parts of the world which are threatened and which we can protect with determination and with the right resources and willpower.'

Listening to Lewis speak can give you goosebumps. In the sea off Bournemouth, those goosebumps battle for supremacy against the goosebumps from how flipping cold the water is. The waves and the current seem to join the battle against me, suddenly the sea's become quite choppy and progress is much slower. But with his words so fresh in my brain, I mean, I can hardly give up can I? Slowly, gruellingly, time and watch vibrations tick over to three hours and I can start heading for home.

Everything becomes easier when I do. Funny that, with the finishing line in sight. More proof that life is simply the story you tell yourself. I'm back where I started with 15 minutes to spare, swim an easy loop out to sea counting down the seconds, and finally exit the water four hours and one minute after I first entered.

My arms and legs have now joined my Transit van feet in the luminous white party. I stagger towards my bag, somehow get some clothes on shivering and a little confused, and head for the car. Hot bot (what we call heated car seats) and a heated steering wheel never felt so good!

At some point on the motorway I realise I'm about to fall asleep. I consider pulling on to the hard shoulder, but fortunately a services sign appears. A mile later, I park in the first available bay and pass out within seconds.

Some indeterminate time later, I wake up when the car reverberates loudly with the sound of an incoming phone call. It's the girls calling from Stockholm in their glad rags and a state of high excitement. They're about to leave for the stadium and Taylor Swift. I'm still in too much of a state to talk. My brain is a 'Blank Space'. I fall back asleep mid-phone call. Swimming... Oh swimming... 'Look What You Made Me Do'.

18

Swimming Fat

I keep being told I have to put weight on to swim the Channel. That I need to add a layer of brown fat to stay warm in the water and avoid hypothermia. And I really don't want to.

Here's the problem. It's taken me more than a decade to drag myself to a place you'd describe as fit and healthy, and scoffing cake for breakfast, ice cream for lunch and chocolate bars before bed – all of which have been recommended to me by various Channel swimming experts – seems completely counterintuitive.

On the day after Jessica Ennis-Hill won heptathlon gold at the London Olympics of 2012, she came to be interviewed on BBC radio. We asked her what's it's like being so fit. The best heptathlete in the world must be in the conversation about being the planet's fittest woman. 'I honestly don't know,' replied Jess. 'I've always been fit, so I've nothing to compare it to.'

Well, I do have something to compare it to. I only started exercising in my 30s when I spotted what looked like a small tube of fat flopping over my belt as I drove to work one day. Vanity led me straight to the gym and a running shoe shop, and I've never looked back. Exercise is a great many things to a great many people and it seems to be all of those things to me. It ticks all of the boxes.

I fell in love with running first and the glorious notion of pushing my limits. A half marathon, a marathon, a marathon in under three hours. A 100-kilometre race, a 100-miler, a multi-day mountain ultra. I once (somehow) completed one of the two hardest foot races on earth, the 153-mile Spartathlon in Greece. On zero training, I found myself on the start line of the hardest 100-miler in the UK, the notorious Arc of Attrition Winter Endurance Race around the rugged coast path of Cornwall. I finished on a broken leg.

I love this stuff. And now I've signed up to swim the Channel, a challenge so far out of my comfort zone it may as well be in a different time zone. But it seems that to complete the challenge, I'll need to get unhealthier and unfitter. It's messing with my brain.

I have another long WhatsApp exchange with Will Ellis, the actor, Channel swimmer and outdoor swim podcaster, who couldn't be kinder or more helpful. Check out this from February, six months ahead of the Channel swim:

> 'After Jersey I lost all my weight by cutting out the liquids and liquid feeds when swimming. Took five weeks and I was back to my fighting weight for pool racing. Give me a ring if you want to know more… it's not difficult IMO. Attached pic is how "big" I got for Round Jersey. Literally about to jump in for nine hours!'

Will then takes me through the exact feeding strategy for his own Channel attempt which will take place a month before I'm hoping to do mine. Every 30 minutes he rotates through three feeds (250ml sucrose-based Maltodextrin with Electrolytes, 250ml Sucrose-based Maltodextrin with Collagen and Ginger cordial, 250ml Fructose-based Maltodextrin).

> 'The idea is that I don't get a drop-off (some call it the Wall) when my sucrose carbs inevitably bottom out and the fructose-based carbs take care of the dip. And treats are vital, for the noodle mainly. I largely use jelly babies. And every 90 minutes I'll have an Ella's Kitchen baby pouch.'

He adds a video of his first feed on his near-record Round Jersey swim. It's like a Formula One pitstop. There's no way I could come close to that sort of speed and professionalism. I watch in awe as his pink swim hat approaches the escort boat behind those powerful shoulders. Almost without breaking stroke Will flips on his back, takes the nutrition bottle from a helpful outstretched arm and chugs the liquid feed, while keeping up momentum by swimming backwards with both legs and his spare arm. No more than five seconds later he's throwing the bottle back towards the boat (it's attached on a line) and swimming off. Equally impressive – and intimidating.

Will manages to look fit and strong despite the extra kilos he's added for the swim. Even on telly, where the camera famously adds its own. And yet still I'm reluctant to put any inches around my own waistline.

In June when David Walliams, who of course smashed his solo swim, chatted to me on air about all things Channel prep, he immediately told me to put on some weight. Will hears the conversation and sends me a WhatsApp.

Friday 7 June 15:22
Will:
Enjoyed your chat with David on the radio… When's your six hour? Did mine last weekend, was fun!
AND PUT ON SOME WEIGHT
Doesn't need to be much, just core warmth.

15:31
Vassos:
Haha! Funny how often I'm hearing that!
Congrats on 6-hour. Got 2x3 in a lake this weekend. Qualifier in late June when I feel ready. Slightly bricking it for now.
Also, Young Woman and the Sea. Film.

15:32

Will:

Except Daisy Ridley wouldn't have survived three hours in the Channel looking like that!!

(Weight comment).

15:33

Vassos:

I'm hoping it's true what they say about not getting much colder after two hours.

15:37

Will:

I hate to burst your bubble there. While it's true one gets used to the cold: assuming temperature remains consistent AND fatigue doesn't set in… but if either one of those changes things can get difficult. Whether you start at night or swim into the night, for example. Another seasoned CW Pro got pulled after three hours last week.

All it takes for a few months is eating chocolate before bed (like, a lot)… which you'll cut out after the fact. The same idea with milkshakes at night and after training. Both of these are easy to remove from your diet and the weight will fall off you. KBO as they say. KBO!!

It's the best part of swimming the Channel!

(I still don't know what KBO means).

The following day I turn up at one of the happiest, most joyful events I've ever had the privilege of attending – and promptly lose all my confidence. It's a 24-hour swim relay around a 500-metre loop of Shepperton Lake. I see this as an opportunity to get in some big-time swim training. I couldn't have it more wrong.

Jenny does the PR for the event and invites me along. On my insistence, she puts me down for two three-hour stints in her team – called 'Alert the Media!' – made up of media types like me. There's always one member of each team in the water, so between us we'll be swimming for 24 hours solid. Everyone else does a single hour here and there, totalling three in total. The swims are non-competitive and nobody is counting how many laps of the lake you manage in your 60 minutes (180 minutes in my case).

There are 500 people in teams of six or eight – and they've all come along to camp, swim, get close to nature, meet like-minded people. All except me. Staying up for 24 hours straight and working on a breakfast show don't go together very well, so I'm going home to sleep between my evening stint and the three hour-swim at dawn the next day. What I end up missing are the glorious hours of darkness, which add another layer of magic to proceedings.

The genius of the event is the decision not to time anyone. And there's no judgement whether you're doing head-down front crawl trying to swim as fast and far as you can (me) or head-up breaststroke having a lovely chat as you go (most other people). Some manage just one lap in their allotted hour, others seven or eight. Nobody cares whether you wear a wetsuit.

Mark Fox invented this glorious celebration of swimming to raise money for the wonderful charity Level Water, which provides swimming lessons for children with disabilities. Around Shepperton Lake there are many prosthetic limbs.

'What we do as a charity is teach disabled kids to swim. Our whole mission is to break down the barriers. Working with pools to give time and space for one-to-one lessons, training their staff, their swim teachers. Level Water means level the playing field so everyone has an opportunity to learn to swim and fall in love with the water – and that's what we wanted our events to be.

'It's not timed. There's no race. The only rule is you've got an hour and then if you want to do one lap, you do one lap, and if you want to do 10 laps, you do 10 laps, but there's nothing else. We've got a team with eight 14- and 15-year-old kids from a school, we've got a team of Ironmen, we've got 70-year-old amputees – all doing the same thing. And it's just inclusive, it's chilled and it's hard. Swimming at 2 a.m. is going to be tricky. And yeah, it's a lovely event. It's not all about being competitive. It's just about doing something as a group, as a community, for a good cause.

'And when we talk about what we do as a charity, a lot of these kids are never going to learn to swim, but some of them might just learn to blow bubbles; that will be the most amazing day of their life. Some of them might learn to do a width; that will be the most amazing day of their life. Some of them will learn to swim and go to the Paralympics. So everyone has their own goal. Everyone has their own Everest. And what this event's allowed people to do is create their own challenge. We don't guide it. We don't force people to do anything other than keep them safe, swim for an hour and then make it what you need it to be.'

Every hour, people crowd around the entry point to the lake and cheer people out of the water, and back in again. There's a wonderful atmosphere of camaraderie and joy. Another truly wonderful thing about the open water occurs to me: it's one of the last places you can be completely disconnected. No-one's on their phone. No-one's watching anything. No-one's engaging in anything but the water and their thoughts. Swimming is a glorious antithesis to our over-comforted, over-convenienced everyday lives. I speak the thought out loud to Mark.

'So when we look at the kids that we teach, the second they jump in, that first moment, there's simply joy all over their face. Even with people like us who've learned to swim from a young age, we jump in this lake and just go, "Wow." Because it's a reset. It's a submersion. It's a total absorption of a different way of life that clears the mind. It makes you feel good. It releases endorphins, releases adrenaline. It's a survival thing as well. If you can't swim, if you don't kick your legs, you'll drown. So there's that element of fear as well that you're doing something to keep yourself alive.

'And swimming in the dark. It is such an abnormal experience, because the fear of what's in front of me, what's below me, what's around me is uncontrollable. How deep is this? What's below? What's there? Everyone has that fear. And what you'll see is from these first two startling buoys, the first night swim, you'll see a lot of very nervous people, and then by the end of that, they'll never want to stop because it takes that disconnect from the world into another level. It's a magical feeling.'

Swimming in the dark is something I'm slowly getting used to with all the Channel training, but you never lose that fear. And day or night, you never lose the sense of disconnect. The longer the swim, the greater the reset. I'm loving this journey. By now my weekly volume is up to around 20 kilometres, mostly in pools squeezed between breakfast shows and school runs. I feel like I've got the fitness; I'm getting the technique; I'm still working on the cold tolerance.

Two weekends previously I had managed four hours in the sea in Bournemouth. The water temperature off the South Coast that day was 14 or 15 degrees, so when my turn comes to dive into Shepperton-on-Thames Lake I'm confident I'll happily handle three hours in much warmer water without having to resort to neoprene. The temperature in the lake is 19 degrees, which is a little warmer than the Channel is expected to be for my solo attempt in September. As I skip through the brightly coloured entry-exit marquee and wade into the water, a woman in a wheelchair is being lowered into the lake beside me and is grinning with sheer pleasure. I smile back at her as I mentally prepare for my triple shift. The water feels fresh and pleasant. I've got this.

And look, I've put the work in. Winter Serpentine swims five mornings a week for three years. Every summer's day has begun with four minutes in 2-degree water courtesy of the ice bath in the garden. Whenever we're in Whitstable, I've revelled in racing into the North Sea to put in the training hours. Days have frequently been organised around tide times. I feel like I've done the acclimatisation and have every reason to be confident.

My body disagrees. During the first lap it seems to take longer than expected to get used to the water temperature. I put it down to the fact that I'm taking it easy and trying to focus on technique. It's still colder than most people would swim in after all.

Meanwhile my goggles are being useless and keep fogging and leaking. I'm constantly having to take them off, empty and rinse. I berate myself for not wearing the new ones. It's hard to get any sort of rhythm. I'm basically having to guess which direction I'm meant to be swimming in, and frequently a member of the safety team paddles up on a kayak and sets me gently back on course. I decide this must be why I'm still feeling so chilly on laps two and three.

Almost half an hour gone and the cold starts to become more of an issue than the crappy goggles. I insist to myself that it's all in my head; remind myself that a fortnight ago I was in 14-degree water and managed to 'firm it'.

This. Is. Not. Cold.

Except, it really is.

My hands and feet are in better shape than they were in the Bournemouth sea, but the rest of me can't stop shivering. People exit the lake after an hour. I'm required to do the same so they can check my number off a list for safety reasons. I briefly consider stopping to put on my wetsuit, but dismiss the thought at once. The ignominy! I dive straight back in.

But now I'm really struggling. I try to stay in the moment, swimming from buoy to buoy on the triangular course, but constantly find reasons to stop. Goggles, needing a wee, resetting my bearings, hoping for any sort of respite from the cold. Only, as I know only too well, it's actually NOT COLD. Most people are wearing wetsuits, but many are not. Few can have put in similar hours to me in recent months.

The second hour seems to last forever. Negative thoughts explode like fireworks against a darkening sky. I remember a primal underwater scream from a recent swim marathon (when my biggest problem was my inability to empty my bladder); it seemed to help. So I let out a scream that probably registers on the Richter Scale in Canada. It only makes things worse.

As a last resort, I try meditating. Counting the breaths, repeating my mantra. Anything to take my mind off the fact that I feel freezing when I surely have no right to feel freezing. This is all in the mind, right? It's the fear of the cold stopping me being able to handle the cold. My brain has become the burden. It's telling me all the things that have gone wrong, and all the things that could still go wrong, and all the things that need to go right for me to be okay.

But, actually, I know I'm already okay. And the reason I'm already okay is that the water is warm (relatively) and I've handled colder for longer. I just need to keep swimming and stop obsessing about the cold. Titanium willpower is all I've got. Zero chance of me giving in to the temptation of neoprene.

After the second hour, I dive for the wetsuit. Jaw frozen open, hands shaking, mind utterly scrambled. I'm so hypothermic I don't even know which are armholes and which are legholes. I attempt to put my left leg into the right arm of the wetsuit. It's two hours into my swim and I still have an hour to go. I don't remember making the decision to exit the lake. It wasn't even a decision. It was an inevitability. It was self-preservation. I head round the corner, hiding from the organisers.

Jenny and Ian from our relay team notice I'm struggling and come rushing over to help. I'm hardly able to speak. Jenny helps me into the wetsuit as Ian feeds me a chocolate biscuit. Good job they don't quite grasp what a state I've got myself into and I'm glad there's no talk of someone else completing my three-hour shift, because I'd probably jump at the chance. I'm consumed by a mixture of gratitude and embarrassment.

After five minutes on land, I'm swimming again. The wetsuit makes all the difference. Within half a lap I'm mentally back in the game and enjoying swimming again. For the time being I push aside thoughts of what the past two hours mean for my Channel attempt and relish the simple pleasure of the front crawl. I become what swim teacher Ray describes as a passenger in my own stroke. I swim a wide line around the buoys so as not to get in anyone's way and power around the course four, five, six, seven times. I'm gutted when the time comes to finish the swim and hand over the baton (actually a pink wristband) to Ian.

The following morning I swim the full three hours in a wetsuit and love every second. As I drive home, I start to consider my options for the Channel. On the one hand, I'm desperate to swim under official rules and have my attempt ratified. One swim hat, one pair of goggles and tight swim shorts only. To do that, it seems I'll definitely have to start taking on board the expert advice and therefore start taking on board the extra calories. And I don't want to. I suspect my mental health would suffer if my diet and physique took a nosedive. The other option is a wetsuit Channel swim and obviously nobody would really mind if I did that. But would I? I'm the guy who muscles through. Wearing a wetsuit would feel like a big old fail.

There's also the safety element to consider. People die in the Channel. Only last year, a strong, fit firefighter from Birmingham vanished while attempting the crossing. A desperate search involving French and Belgian military helicopters, plus navy and police patrol boats, was eventually called off when the body of Ian Hughes washed up in Belgium. The father-of-two was raising money for three charities when he lost sight of the boat. While asking for privacy, his family said their lives were shattered. I owe it to my family, and also to all the people who've been offering help and guidance, to take this endeavour as seriously as it deserves. This is proper.

I do a lot of soul searching. Outwardly I pretend it's a light conundrum, but inwardly I'm struggling. Quite honestly, the idea of putting on weight horrifies me. Equally, having fallen in love with the wonderful world of channel swimming, I want to honour these superstars by fully respecting the challenge.

One argument swings it. My friend Chris reminds me on air one morning that what I most love is going outside my comfort zone. And what could be further outside my comfort zone than putting on some fat? So, as the Queen of France Marie Antoinette famously (if apocryphally) said when told that her starving peasants had no bread, 'Let them eat cake.' I start eating lots of cake.

19

Swimming Sixties

'Congratulations on being awesome!' As first questions go, it's not going to win any journalism awards, is it? But I literally can't help myself. And I do have previous.

I once interviewed the tennis player Johanna Konta live on the BBC. It was the morning after she'd been knocked out in the semi-finals of Wimbledon by the great Venus Williams. She'd just been given a grilling on the *Today* programme on Radio 4. Nothing against the *Today* programme, it's what they do. Find the news line. Ask the hard questions. 'Are you even British?' the Aussie-born British number one was asked (despite the fact she'd already represented Team GB at the Olympics). Konta then came on our show, nervous a repeat might be on the way. But she'd charmed her way through the Wimbledon draw, even finding time to share pictures of her baking exploits. So all I could think to start the interview with was: 'I hope it's okay, but we absolutely love you Jo!'

The same thing is now happening with Diana Nyad. It's 9 p.m. in the UK and, after dozens of emails to her advisors and agents, I've finally managed to persuade a true legend of open water swimming to have a chat for this book. *Nyad*, the movie of her seemingly impossible swim from Cuba to Florida, has just been nominated for an Oscar. She has another Netflix documentary, *The Other Side*, in production. And she's had to deal with criticism from some sections of the marathon-swim community who continue to raise concerns about the validity of her record-breaking swim. Questions about whether all the rules were followed to the letter. (See the Appendix on p. 199 for the full rules.) Personally, I don't really care about any of that. What is undeniable is the sheer magnitude of the achievement. And the inspiration she's given countless others.

Diana Nyad was already one of the world's great open water swimmers by the time she hit 25. She broke records including Round Manhattan (28 miles, 7 hours 57 minutes) and Gulf of Naples (22 miles, 8 hours 11 minutes). Then in 1978, aged 28, she attempted the unprecedented swim between Cuba and Florida, from Havana to Key West. It is 110 miles of insane currents, tropical storms and deadly box jellyfish, all with the constant threat of attack from beneath by sharks. After fighting a losing battle for almost 42 hours and 76 miles, team doctors removed her from the water amid strong winds and currents pushing her off-course towards Texas.

She promptly gave up swimming and became a sportscaster. And then, on her 60th birthday, which is when the film begins, she began to wonder… What if? She promptly began training again and, astonishingly, decided to give Cuba to Florida another shot in 2011 aged 61: 'Because I'd like to prove to the other 60-year-olds that it is never too late to start your dreams.' High winds again put paid to her attempt and she was reluctantly pulled from the water after 29 hours.

So she tried again. And after 41 hours, more adverse weather and several box jellyfish stings that caused her to struggle to breathe and could have killed her, she failed again. So she tried again. Two storms, many gruelling miles and more jellyfish stings later, she was forced to abandon once more.

So she tried again. On the morning of 31 August 2013, Diana began her fifth bid to swim from Cuba to Florida. And 53 hours later, at 1:55 p.m. on 2 September, her hand touched the sand on Smathers Beach in Key West. Her faltering steps took her clear of the water and she collapsed into the embrace of her team.

She had three things to tell the friendly mob of onlookers who'd gathered to watch her achieve a lifelong dream. Her slurred remarks were received with roars and cheers: 'One is, we should never ever give up. Two is, you're never too old to chase your dreams. Three is, it looks like a solitary sport, but it's a team.' She was then taken away on a stretcher.

I felt I'd gone through something of a feat of endurance when I finally got to chat to Diana on the phone. She's a busy woman, a force of nature, she rarely gives interviews. It had taken three months, dozens of emails and Nyad-like tenacity. I am thrilled to finally get the chance to speak with her at 9 p.m. and approaching my bedtime in London, lunchtime on the west coast of the USA.

Me:

'Congratulations on being awesome!'

Diana:

'Well, this is my pleasure. Thank you for the opportunity. I must say that my agent and I were just laughing as we are not 100% sure if your first name is Alexander or is that your last name?'

Me:

'The last name is Alexander. My first name is Vassos.'

Diana:

'It is Vassos, so where does that come from? I am not familiar with that name, Vassos.'

Me:

'It's a Greek name, actually. I'm named after my grandfather who was Vassos Hippocrates, which is a fantastic name. I just got Vassos Alexander.'

Diana:

'Well, I like it. You know my Greek heritage as well, and my father's name was Aristotle, so it's not that far from where you are there.'

Me:

'Aristotle and Hippocrates and Diana. Thank you for taking the time to speak to me. As I say, I'm so excited. And I suppose the first question I have for you is how do you face down what is on the face of it an impossible challenge and decide to go for it anyway?'

Diana:

'It's such a deep question, Vassos, because we could say, well, whose definition of impossible is it? If I said to you today at age 74 that I'd never played the French horn in my life, but Vassos, I'm going to today, on 1 February 2024, take up the French horn and my goal in 10 years is to play for the New York Philharmonic, to sit in first chair French horn for the New York Philharmonic. Well, I think both of us could say you don't have to be a naysayer or pessimistic to say that is not going to happen.

'It's not just highly unlikely, it is not going to happen. I have no background, I have no talent, it's not going to happen. Whereas to pick, as an open water swimmer who's held many records around the world, to pick a swim that, on the face of it, has seemed to be impossible for several other very good swimmers, and could be called impossible by many, that's very different.

'And then let's get philosophical and let's get Greek with our Greek background, both of us, and talk about the whole notion of the journey being what life is all about. It's not the destination. We're not hoping to get to best. What we're hoping to do is take a journey in everything we do, whether it's raising a child or taking on a business, or entering and engaging with full commitment in a sporting event. If you don't like the training, if you don't like the planning, if you don't like the commitment to who you have to become every single day to get to your destination, then you are on the wrong journey.

'For me, after failing – and I hate to use that word, because there were epic adventures in the ocean, all those four times before I made it across – but when I came to make the journey for the fifth time, it was because the members of that team and I weren't done. We had not reached the destination.

'But you know what? In some ways, to be absolutely candid, that wasn't what it was all about. It was being together and gathering more intel, more science, more understanding of what's out there. Can we be the smart team? The brave team? Can we be the prepared team? Can we be maybe the lucky team? Can we be the ones to finally make this crossing?

'I know I'm going on and on about what seemed to be a simple question. How does one face the impossible? Well, to me, it was never impossible. It was something I thought

I was capable of and my team thought we were capable of, but that doesn't mean that anybody else in the world thought we were. Yeah, it was difficult.

'I do think also that it's inspiring to have the courage to fail. It's easy if the bar is set low and you can do something very well, whether it's academic or athletic or anything, but then what do you learn about yourself in trying to reach that very low bar? Almost nothing. It's something you could do with your eyes closed. You don't know what your potential is. You don't know what your talents are.

'But if you set that bar high, something may be impossible, or shall we say close to impossible, but now you are going to drill down into all your potential. Every aspect of your being is going to be called upon. You may not get there, but the journey will be worthwhile. But the point is, no matter what that journey, you are going to be in a state of discovery about the outside world and about your inner world, and who you are and how you must evolve your thinking.'

Me:

'I love that the journey is the destination. I was lucky enough to know Sir Roger Bannister, who is well known in athletics circles. He was the first human being to run the mile in under four minutes. He said to me that every day you should try and get outside of your comfort zone. Every day. Because then that comfort zone expands and expands and expands. I guess in your case, Diana, your comfort zone is just that much bigger than the rest of ours.'

Diana:

'When I go to sleep every night, I do a quick accounting. I say, "I'm never going to get to live that day again. What did

I do with that day? Do I look back with regret on that day?" Because simple as it sounds, the way you choose to live today is the way you've chosen to live your life.

'With all due respect to Roger Bannister if he wants to go beyond his comfort zone every single day, because every individual deserves to go about their lives as they want to, but for me it's not about that. It's going to sleep each night and making that measurement. Saying to myself, "I just couldn't have done anything I could be more satisfied with, more proud of, more happy with, than what I did with that day."

'Now, does that always mean I'm on the cusp of doing something outrageous? It could be I'm taking my dog at sunrise to the beach to stare across the horizon and think about this planet and think about the Stephen Hawking book that I read the night before and watch the joy of my dog sprinting up and down in the surf. Is that a good way to spend at least a couple of hours in a day? In my definition, yes. Did it take me beyond any comfort zone? No, not at all. But I want to go to bed saying, "I have no regrets about that day."'

Me:

'What a great philosophy. What keeps you motivated, Diana? When you've accomplished something so epic, so groundbreaking, so wonderful, what keeps you motivated? I can hear from how you're speaking what a positive person you are, what a deep thinker you are. What keeps you that way?'

Diana:

'Look at me. I got to come back at an older age, in my 60s, to be involved at a world-class level in this sport. Not all athletes can. Most football players, whether it be American football or European football, you're probably not going to play well into your 70s, are you? You're probably not going to have that explosive speed and strength again. But for endurance sports, if you want to climb Everest or snowshoe across Antarctica or swim from Cuba to Florida, it's very possible with the right training, the right attitude, the right discipline, the right team.

'Most people are in their 20s or 30s when they really do their world-class stuff. Even though they will know deep love, maybe they will have children, they'll have partners, they'll have lifetime experiences, they'll live great lives, because of the nature of sports they will probably never, ever have that drama again. It could be that Serena Williams... I'm not going to comment on Serena Williams' life. It could be that she's wildly happy and she doesn't miss the highlights of tennis at all, but I would imagine she's never going to feel that particular high octane of playing in front of thousands of people adored by millions worldwide on the nighttime match at the US Open Final. I doubt she's ever going to feel that kind of adrenaline again.

'I'm not comparing myself to Serena Williams. I'm just saying that even though I got the chance to be older and have this feeling, when I walked out on that beach in Key West after swimming for 53 non-stop hours, I doubt I'm going to feel that rush, that high, again. But that doesn't mean I can't live a deep life that is filled, as I said before, with chasing big dreams, having the courage to fail and going to bed at night and believing I've just done everything with that day. That doesn't mean that I can't have all that.

'Also, I'll tell you that I'm nothing special. I've had a chance to travel all around the world. Sometimes I could hold the globe and say, "My God, I've been in the interior of Borneo. I've been swimming with whales down in the southern oceans of Patagonia below the Antarctic circle line. I've done this and that. I've been here and there and met all these people." I do believe that everybody – I think it's part of the human condition – that we all have special traits. We all have courage, although I don't think that we're called upon to display a lot of what the human being is in modern life anymore.

'But I know for me, I think one thing somewhat unusual about me, Vassos, was that before double digits, when I was eight, nine years old, I was already very aware of the loud ticking of the clock. I was already all freaked out that this life, this special thing that the Pulitzer Prize-winning poet Mary Oliver calls our one wild and precious life, I knew it was going to be short. I knew I'd better not waste any time. I'd better get thinking about who I wanted to be, what I wanted to do. How was I going to get there? What kind of people was I going to surround myself with?

'I've been very focused my whole life on how fast this thing goes by. Now at the age of 74, believe me the clock is ticking louder than it's ever ticked before. I'm still vital. I've got a lot of energy, I have a lot of dreams, and I bet for the next 20 years I'll be pushing hard and living hard. It'll all be good. But I think that for me a lot of the emphasis, the motivation, comes from knowing how special this life is and knowing how short it is.'

Me:

'That really strikes a chord with me. I've felt the same way since a very young age. I have no doubt that in two decades' time you'll still be as positive and energetic as I can hear you are today. Can you share any rituals or routines that you follow?'

Diana:

'Well, I think the most important one... I'm not going to pretend this has been every single day of my life. Sometimes you're in extreme circumstances. But as a general rule, most of my life I've gotten up before the sun. It started with being a little swimmer, a little awkward six-, seven-year-old swimmer. It continues as a funny thing. I do it as a moment of humour, really, but in front of audiences if I'm giving a little talk or presentation, I play a couple of bars on the bugle, and I'm known for this, of "Reveille", because people know it.

'All around the world, we know those notes. That means get up. The sun is about to rise. You'd better get up before the sun. You'd better not miss the dawn. You don't want to miss your life. And so for me, it's been important to. Some days, as I said, you can't. Some days you've been up for two or three days doing something. You're travelling, you're jet lagged, you have appointments. But if I'm living a day that I have a lot of choice over, I get up before the sun. I play the 'Reveille' (much to the dismay of my neighbours) on my bugle and I just dive into a pretty extreme exercise routine right away. Other days I'm rushing to catch a flight, but I want to get up with the dawn. I want to embrace the day.

'I've been reading. Not in any – believe me – mathematical, scientific, astrophysical way, but I've been reading about the cosmos ever since I've been a teenager and had this more emotional, philosophical appreciation of this little blue speck, this little blue spot, as the brilliant Carl Sagan put it, that we live on. How lucky we are that we were, with the Big Bang, just catapulted into this little circle of orbit around this particular sun at this distance to have this much warmth, but not too much heat, to develop carbon enough to develop life.

There may be other life like this if the universe exists unto infinity, but as far as we know in this part of the universe we are the only ones that got this lucky.

'I have disappointments, I have arguments with people, I have down moments, et cetera, but mostly I try to look out and think about reading Stephen Hawking, reading Carl Sagan, and thinking about this universe and this Earth that we live on.

'That brings us to the marathon swimming and 1875 was the first English Channel swim. Captain Matthew Webb. Ever since people have been reading stories of open water swimming and all of the gruelling stuff comes in. It's so cold, it's so rough, it's so long. Its sensory deprivation is extreme, the sleep deprivation is extreme, it takes a toll on the body.

'On the other hand, I like to try to remember and to tell people that there's also awe. That to be out 50, 60 miles from the coast and be travelling over the curvature of the earth with your own stroke, the power of your own trained body, to be travelling, to look up and to see two billion stars literally in the middle of a clear night in summer above the Gulf Stream, a lot of it is very majestic. It's very inspiring. I don't think I could ever have those same feelings anywhere else except out in the ocean. What I'm immersed in and in love with is this blue dot of Planet Earth, but particularly from the ocean point of view.'

Me:

'I think that might be my favourite ever answer to a question I've asked. Thank you very much for that. I've only got one more, I promise. How has your life changed since the film came out? Because it seems everybody on Earth has seen the film now.'

Diana:

'We're lucky it has at points trended, and I use that verb in a fictional way, because I honestly don't even know what it means. But it has trended number one in the world on Netflix on and off over the past few months. Millions of people have seen it from China to Chile to Wyoming. Bonnie [Stoll, portrayed by Jodie Foster in the film] and I have heard from thousands and thousands of people who are inspired by the grit of this character, my character, by my character's unapologetic approach to her dreams, by the friendship of these two women who are just in it together. Nothing will get in their way. I'm very proud of it.

'But that's us. I'm a grounded person and so is Bonnie. We are honoured. We are deeply, deeply honoured that these actresses decided to play these roles, that this writer and this production team and these directors took on this movie, that Netflix put all this money behind it and believed that people needed to hear this story.

'I'm deeply honoured, but does it change my life? Yeah, I'm a public speaker and do I maybe get a few more gigs and do I get paid a bit more at least for the next few months while the movie's name is out? Yes, but that doesn't change my life. I have the way I want to live my life and my goals in front of me. This movie was just a phantasmagoric moment for both me and Bonnie. We are so grateful for it. We can barely believe that it came true for us and we have to pinch ourselves. But our lives, our day-to-day who we are, what we want to do, that hasn't changed one iota. It's just a moment of celebration.

'But this movie hasn't changed my life. I've learned early on with just little bouts of... I even hate to use the word fame. It sounds so pretentious, but little bouts of notoriety. You don't want to make the mistake of thinking that when someone comes up to you in an airport saying, "Oh, are you Diana Nyad? Can I get a selfie?" that you are being loved or you are even being deeply admired.

'When I get notes from a man who has Parkinson's and says that he's close to giving up and he saw this movie and his wife thought, they thought together, "I'm still me. Maybe I can't button my shirt anymore, but I'm still me. I'm going to be me the best I can till the day I die." If that's happening out there, then that is huge and it affects me. It affects deeply my inner self, but it doesn't change my life. I can't depend on people admiring me or people knowing about me as the cornerstone of my values. You know what I mean? We will be forgotten very quickly once this movie's done and the next year's movies are out. It's just been, let's just say, a magical moment.'

Me:

'Well, Diana, I was right. You are 100% awesome. Honestly, I think if you set your mind to it, you could play the French horn in any orchestra in the world.'

20

Swimming Downhill VI

When Ray started helping with my swim stroke and mentioned the phrase 'swimming downhill', it gave me something to aim for, but in all honesty I doubted I'd get there. However, I put the work in, did the drills, and swimming downhill is actually the best way to describe what ploughing through the water now feels like. Even on a very long swim, to use another of Ray's phrases, you're just a passenger in your stroke. Simultaneously, you're swimming faster than before and expending less effort.

So I reckon it's probably a good idea to ask Ray for some general advice that everyone can benefit from, because the swim stroke is relatively easy to master if you break it down. The catch, the kick, the stroke. And first and foremost, before you move on to anything else, you've got to master the breathing. Over to you, Ray:

'Actually that's not the case. I see lots of excellent endurance athletes. And pretty much all of them say "Just sort my breathing out. It's my breathing, it's my breathing." But in my opinion, you cannot achieve rhythmic, confident breathing without a rhythmic, confident, efficient stroke. You simply can't.

'So I teach the stroke first and then move on to the breathing. Because if the stroke is lopsided and asymmetrical, and there's no rhythm to it, and there's a degradation and the swimmer gets tired, how on earth are they going to work on their breathing? So some people find it strange, but I actually go quite a long way down the line with the stroke before I turn my attention to the ins and outs of breathing.

'With a lot of swimmers, the thing is trying to get them to slow down. Even if an excellent swimmer comes to see me, and plenty of excellent swimmers do, they still plateau. So slow down, isolate the movements in drill form and think about your stroke.

'I had a chat with the World 10K champion Sharon van Rouwendaal recently. She was planning her career after the Paris Olympics and she left me a WhatsApp voice message, as youngsters do these days. And she said, "Oh I'm happy to come over to your pool and do a demonstration." And the first word she used to describe her stroke was long.

'Now, if you keep your head still and you extend, you will also rotate. So if you imagine with your head still, you reach forward, your body's obviously horizontal. If you reach forward, you'll extend and you will rotate. So that's the extension and rotation of the stroke. But most people struggle, because when they breathe, they basically try and climb out the water to one degree or another.

'So not only do you need to train yourself to extend and rotate or keep the stroke long to begin with, you also need to breathe around that platform of extension and rotation. Once you have that platform, that rhythmic platform, then you can start delving down into the nuances of the catch, the kick and even the breathing. It's always, always about the basics.

'The catch is essentially engaging the water with a large effective paddle as early as possible. Your paddle goes from the crook of your elbow to the tip of your fingertips.

And essentially what you're trying to do is get that facing backwards as early as possible.

'It is something that elite swimmers appear to do and the rest of us struggle with, but it's quite simple. Once you've learned the movement, you repeat it, you cement it, you get used to applying the power later. But basically, in one sentence, you're trying to get a large surface area facing backwards as early as possible.

'Simply put, the back of the stroke is just pushing through to the end. And talking about extending, keeping the stroke long. You're long at the front and you're long at the back, certainly when you're learning to swim. Often people become so obsessed with engaging the water, catching the water, they forget about the back of the stroke. But the catch actually doesn't make you a faster swimmer. It's what you do once you've got hold of the water and you need to push down past the waistline.'

'The long distance leg kick is very different to a sprinter's leg kick. I always use Katie Ledecky as an example, because she's world-class from 200 to 1500 metres. She's unbeatable at 1500 metres. Hasn't lost a race in 15 years. And the way she kicks in the 1500 metres is completely different to the way she kicks in the 200 metres. The 200 metres, it's a muscular, powerful eight feet leg kick. Eight kicks per cycle of the arm to speed her down the pool.

'The two beat long-distance kick is very much a driver of the rotation. What I taught Vassos was a hip-driven stroke rather than a shoulder-driven stroke, because he was a late comer to swimming and had more of a runner's physique, and that kick added power to that rotation and acceleration to the stroke. There was a little bit of propulsion and that put the top hat on his body position. That's what the long-distance leg kick is. Some people get it really easily, some people really struggle. But it's worth the journey, as with anything in life.

'I'm lost without my two beat leg kick. If I wear a wetsuit in a 10K swim, I go the same speed as I do without the wetsuit. Shorter distances, I'd go faster in a wetsuit, because it's more about power. In long distance swimming, I miss that leg kick so much that I'm the same speed. That leg kick is such an integral part of the stroke.

'With breathing, the trick is to exhale fully beneath the water. And as I said, if you've got that rhythmic, confident, efficient stroke, then it's a lot easier. In fact, it's essential in my opinion. But the fact is you need to get the air out under the water. And what I encourage people to do is – I give them a midway between constant exhalation and holding it and letting it go. And then they tend to find their way. It's just basically exhaling beneath the water, but if you haven't got that rhythmic, confident, efficient stroke, you subconsciously or even consciously limit your exhalation. You don't want to lose control.'

21

Swimming Poo

Sod's law is definitely a thing. No sooner have I gleefully announced to a thousand people that I've not been remotely ill during my open water swimming journey, than I instantly succumb.

I've been swimming in the Serpentine in Hyde Park for almost a decade, in the tidal Thames in South West London since before the first lockdown, and in the North Sea in Whitstable since 2020. I'm aware of all the duck mites in the Serpentine. They can result in something horrible called swimmer's itch or cercarial dermatitis, a skin rash caused by an allergic reaction to parasites found in duck poo. And of course I know that water companies use the latter two as dumping grounds for their overflow sewage. But I am careful.

For instance, I would be sure to rinse after swimming in the Serpentine during mite season. And then there's the Thames: highest risk IMO. There used to be an X account that let you know when and where Thames Water would discharge into the river, and I always refused to swim for a week afterwards. Where we live in Barnes, we're right between the two worst offenders, Mogden Sewage Treatment Works and Hammersmith Pumping Station, so most of the swimmers I know tend to be extra cautious (although there are some who'll cheerfully swim again after just one tide). These are the sort of messages we used to dread:

'@ThamesCSOAlerts: Rower notification from Thames Water: Hammersmith Pumping Station (PS). Following the recent rainfall, Hammersmith Pumping Station has in the last hour discharged heavily diluted storm water into the River Thames, due to a lack of capacity in the existing sewer network...'

or

'@ThamesCSOAlerts: Rower Notification from Thames Water: Mogden Sewage Treatment Works (STW). Following the recent rainfall, Mogden Sewage Treatment Works will in the next hour discharge heavily diluted storm water into the River Thames. Storm water is screened, settled in tanks and mixed with...'

Always those ominous three dots to finish... And always the mild irritation that only rowers merit a mention. The X account was receiving the discharge emails from Thames Water and repeating them for us on X. The dots probably meant they'd run out of characters, but in my head the dots were Twitter speak for the asterisks in s**t. Storm discharges invariably contain raw sewage. Since the launch of their online map in 2023, Thames Water have stopped sending discharge emails, so @ThamesCSOAlerts is now defunct, which is a real shame. Somehow it was always easier to check a feed than an online map before swimming. These days I'm often swimming in the Thames on guesswork.

Which may be why I came down with E. coli the day after telling a field full of a thousand people how safe open water swimming is. I was on stage at an adventure festival alongside far more qualified people for a swimming panel – world open water champion Keri-Anne Payne and *Outdoor Swimmer* founder Simon Griffiths.

Somebody asked about water pollution. Simon and Keri-Anne both answered fulsomely and sensibly and advised on what precautions to take before swimming. I then waxed lyrical about not overthinking, enjoying the moment, communing with nature, the buzz you get from the cold water, just generally not worrying about it and diving in. In all my time in the Thames and the North Sea, I concluded gleefully, I'd never so much as suffered from an upset tummy. I then cheerfully threw in the truism about drinking Coke after a swim.[1]

The following day, ALL the symptoms: diarrhoea, stomach cramps, mild fever, blood in the stools. In the previous four days, despite recent rainfall, I'd swum for an hour in the Thames and for two hours in the North Sea in Kent. My instinct told me the sea was to blame. Should've gone to SOS Whitstable.

For Thames Water in London, read Southern Water in Kent. Whenever they discharge into the North Sea, the Instagram account @soswhitstable kicks in. They're very active, publishing pictures of the sewage, testing water pollution, letting everyone know whenever there's been a dump. And here's why they bother: go to their Insta and you'll see glorious pictures of the Kentish coastline under blue skies, the sea looking ravishing and inviting and swimmers taking full advantage, along with a pinned post:

'SOSwhitstable: We absolutely love where we live and want to protect this. These photos sum up why we started SOS

---

[1] There's an often-cited (and possibly apocryphal) story about a triathlon in Buckinghamshire after which every competitor fell ill except those who'd drunk a can of full-fat Coke after the swim.

Whitstable. In the 9 days since 1st November there has been over 103 hours of releases from one outfall alone in this catchment area. Was it safe to go in? Who knows. Did we swim properly? Not a chance. Losing this amazing amenity is heartbreaking for us. Even more so the knock-on effect of this environmental disaster on our fishing industry and local economy. We will continue to make this better. Love wins, right?'

SOS Whitstable liaise with other water quality campaign groups to put together petitions and pile pressure on to the water companies and the government. And they organise mass protests. In October 2022 thousands of people, including the local MP and several celebrities, descended on Whitstable beach to 'turn it into a crime scene.' Feargal Sharkey and Paul Whitehouse are chief supporters. Before the speeches and the music, everybody linked arms to barricade the beach while a loud siren wailed and a series of damning statistics were read out about Southern Water's awful record on sewage pollution. The crime scene theme was a nod to the continuing releases into the sea.

SOS Whitstable volunteers frequently wade into that sea to test the water quality and post the results. Ed Acteson is their spokesperson:

'I'm from Herne Bay originally, so I've swum in the sea my entire life. But during the lockdown was the first time I started going in all year round. And of course when you start swimming outside of the bathing season, that's when you become aware of the problem, because that is when the majority of releases happen. And Whitstable has a passionate year-round swimming community.

'SOS Whitstable began during the first lockdown, because obviously people weren't able to access gyms or sports clubs or any sort of social venue either. So in Whitstable people were turning to the beach and swimming as an excuse to go outside, meet people and get some exercise. Wild swimming was really taking off. And as people got involved, suddenly awareness about things like sewage pollution increased, too. And we realised there was a real problem.

'Rosie Duffield, who is our local MP, hosted a public meeting in Whitstable with representatives from Southern Water and the Environment Agency. And effectively we were totally underwhelmed with their responses to the scale of the problem and the risk to public health. We didn't feel like anyone was really taking it seriously enough or that enough action was going to be taken. So we decided to form SOS Whitstable.

'Initially it started off just as a group of friends who swim together. We were just going to try to put some pressure on Southern Water to stop the issue locally. And since then, obviously, with things like our petition and our protest, it's escalated a bit and we've become more on the national agenda.'

I've joined them on the beaches. And I've joined them on the streets (in Teddington). The atmosphere on a mass protest is simultaneously furious and amicable, a heady mix.

In west London Thames Water are trying to push through a plan to extract millions of litres of fresh water from the river and replace them with millions of litres of sewage. The Save Our Lands and River campaign has been supported by all local river users (rowers, sailors, paddle boarders, swimmers) as well as over a hundred local businesses. We're making a loud enough noise and we're being heard. It's also quite fun being interviewed for the news.

The *Times* newspaper has started a 'Clean It Up' campaign of its own. The BBC have become involved – reporting that United Utilities repeatedly dumped millions of litres of raw sewage illegally into Lake Windermere between 2021 and 2023, and failed to declare it. The problem is urgent. Water companies are only allowed to release untreated sewage when it rains heavily to stop homes flooding. But, as the BBC reported, this has frequently been done prematurely, saving the water companies millions of pounds. According to the Environment Agency, sewage spills more than doubled in 2023 – from 1.75 million hours in 2022 to 3.6 million hours in 2023.

Sir Keir Starmer vowed to end the sewage scandal when he replaced Rishi Sunak as Prime Minister in July 2024. And in September 2024 it was announced that water company bosses could be banned from receiving bonuses and even sent to prison under government legislation to combat pollution.

So we're being heard and the pressure is working, but the campaigns can be a double-edged sword, especially in Whitstable. The town is synonymous with oysters, fishing and hospitality. All those are massively impacted by the sewage, but the more campaigners spotlight the issue, the more they're potentially contributing to Whitstable having a reputation as a sewage hotspot. Ed again:

'The problem is, as with any situation, sticking your head in the sand isn't the solution. The way to fix this issue is to solve it, to improve how we treat sewage. And then the quality of oysters and fish and bathing will improve and that will long-term be beneficial to Whitstable.

'Southern Water have become very controlling about our water testing, even though we're using kits that they recommended and provided. They've disputed results, they've said we're not allowed to publish data and they've tried to make us sign a contract saying that we won't talk about any of the results publicly unless we go through them first. And it's obviously problematic, because we're all unpaid volunteers doing this in our spare time on top of our careers and families and social lives.

'It's just a classic example of Southern Water trying, in my view, to hide what they're doing. I've literally just done a Twitter thread today about how they have been hiding releases on their interactive map and there's one down in Rye, which they've classed as non-impacting. So they haven't displayed it on their map and it's been going on for 200 hours. I mean there's just all sorts of different shenanigans designed to mitigate the scrutiny they get and hide the impacts of what they're doing. And I suppose a large part of our job is just constantly trying to find and expose that.

'Whereas in recent years you've had so many really divisive issues like Brexit that have polarised people and led to some quite aggressive arguments, almost everyone is united on this issue – that pumping sewage into watercourses is a terrible idea and that we shouldn't do it. And as far as I'm concerned, the only people that take a different approach to that are people who stand to benefit from it in some way, whether it's a political party like the Conservatives who are effectively not wanting to regulate this issue or the water companies who profit from polluting.

'The tide is definitely turning but it is difficult to say how long it's going to be like that. I mean, a few years ago the big issue was plastic in the ocean. Now the narrative, as far as the news is concerned, has changed. And you hear far less about plastic and far more about sewage pollution. So from our point of view, the risk is the news cycle will move on and they'll find something else to focus on.

'But engagement on our social feeds is unreal. We've only got 7000 followers but we'll tweet something and get hundreds of thousands of responses. Most companies would kill for that level of engagement. It shows how many people are really passionate about this and yeah, I think as long as it stays in the public narrative, eventually it's going to contribute to political change if not fixing the issue.

'So we're just going to keep going with it and if we're still doing it in 10 years, we're still doing it in 10 years. But we would hope it would be less than that at the very least, we can say we played a part in helping keep sewage in Whitstable down.'

The other big worry, of course, is the fact that the pollution is putting people off going in the water. This is Simon who was on that panel with me, from *Outdoor Swimmer* magazine. He lives right by the Thames in Teddington and, quite apart from being able to gauge how popular the sport is by how many copies of the magazines he sells, he can see from his sitting room window how many people turn up for their Saturday morning dip:

'There was this booming interest in outdoor swimming through the pandemic. The growth has flattened off, but there's still a big latent interest. Where we do have a huge challenge at the moment is around water quality.

'So the amazing campaigning that SOS and others have done, Feargal Sharkey being at the forefront, they have done an amazing job of putting sewage pollution on to the political agenda. But it's also created a massive wave of anxiety among people who already swim, and people who are considering swimming, about their safety in open water. And I can see that it's a threat to event organisers, because people are saying, "Well, how can you guarantee that your event is going to be safe?" And it's a threat to the whole concept of swimming outside in nature.'

Simon is bang on about this. Unless people can feel confident in the water quality, they will be hesitant about swimming in it. And it definitely takes the edge off the enjoyment if you're thinking, 'This is nice, but I might be sick tomorrow.' Until recently, there was one official bathing place in the whole of the Thames, Wolvercote Mill Stream. Now it's so full of E. coli it's lost that status. So whereas people used to say, 'You are mad swimming in there, it's so cold,' they now say, 'You are mad swimming in there, it's polluted.'

The women's and men's triathlons at the Paris Olympics had to be delayed due to pollution in the River Seine. And the French authorities had spent billions of Euros to make the water safe to swim in. It was the same story with the open water swimming at the Games. And even the 2024 Oxford-Cambridge Boat Race, Putney to Mortlake on the exact stretch of the Thames where I live, was affected. Crews were advised not to enter the water due to elevated levels of E. coli. The Oxford rowers still got sick and lost a race they'd been expected to win. One of the crew put it rather well after the race, with typical Oxford understatement: 'It would have been ideal not to have so much poo in the water.'

22

Swimming USA

I've mentioned this before, but it never ceases to amaze. Time does somersaults when you swim. Same sort of thing happens on a very long run, but in the water it's more acute. You have nothing to look at or listen to, just your stroke and your thoughts for company. Some minutes seem to take an hour. Many hours pass by in seconds. That last bit is what I'm counting on as I slip into the dark waters of Lake Tahoe in California before dawn one Monday morning. I'm planning an eight-hour training swim, my longest by far. The sheer weight of minutes – 480! – is intimidating. I've run continuously for four times as long, but only swum for half that time. My goggles don't seem to fit properly and need adjusting every few minutes. I don't think it's the goggles, though. I think it's nerves. I'm properly daunted by the task I've set myself.

And the other issue is, while the hours will hopefully slip by unnoticed once the goggles behave themselves and I finally start swimming properly, back on land a lot of life goes by in eight hours. Especially when you're in the middle of a family trip around the USA National Parks. I'm testing my wife's patience, I can tell. Two days ago was the Alcatraz swim, which finished later than planned. Then yesterday, coincidentally, was the San Francisco Marathon.

I'm not sure Caroline believes that I didn't know it was happening until a fortnight ago when I saw a woman wearing the previous year's finishers' tee-shirt. 'San Francisco Marathon: 7.23.23' it said. The numbers grazed my eyes for a second until I worked out that the day and month were the American way round. Which got me thinking, oh that's late July… I wonder… And as luck would have it, the 2024 marathon did indeed coincide with our 48 hours in San Francisco. Actually, I can see Caroline's point: I'm not sure I even believe myself. But the fact is, being me, once I knew it was happening, I could hardly *not* enter.

So, two nights in San Francisco, one Alcatraz swim, one hilly marathon, and now we're about to enjoy the first of three days in South Lake Tahoe and I'm disappearing off on an eight-hour training swim. With exactly the same planned for tomorrow. My wife is a saint. Yesterday we sat down to plan the following two days and I noticed both mornings were free. So seizing my opportunity between mountain hikes, as if rolling under a descending metal shutter commando-style, I arranged these two big swims. At least I'll be done before lunch, so a sort of compromise. In my defence, Channel attempts do involve a LOT of training. And I promise that these are absolutely the last big swims of the holiday (until we reach Lake Powell).

It's 4 a.m. as I enter the water, which is cool but not cold, pleasantly refreshing and much warmer than San Francisco Bay – despite being 6225 feet above sea level. That's roughly double the height of Scafell Pike, the tallest mountain in England. I have no idea how a lake can fail to be freezing at this altitude. And such a big lake too. Lake Tahoe is almost half a mile deep in places. If you drained the lake and poured the contents on to an area the size of the UK, you'd cover the entire British Isles in almost a metre of water. In North America, only the five Great Lakes are larger.

I'm starting the swim in the dark both for the sake of marital harmony and to get me used to swimming at night, which I may have to do crossing the English Channel. The dark definitely adds a layer of toughness. Shadowy peaks loom ominously all around and I have no idea what sort of creatures lurk below. Vast swathes of the shoreline are uninhabited, with the occasional exception of a campsite, marina or hotel. Dark and isolated here really does mean dark and isolated. Barely half an hour in and this swim is already testing the limits of my fortitude.

Once it gets light, Lake Tahoe will be the most brilliant blue. That's what I focus on as I continue swimming apprehensively anti-clockwise, hugging the shore. Just swim until dawn, about two hours, then turn back the way you came and enjoy the beauty. I've left snacks on the shore where we're staying. Just manage four hours in the water, then a swift, standing breakfast, and four hours after that I'll be done.

Even in the dark, the water is amazing. Lake Tahoe is one of the most pure bodies of water anywhere in the world, with 99.994% purity. You can genuinely drink it – and I do. Commercially distilled water is 99.998% pure.

Somehow I don't feel tired despite two active days in San Francisco. My stroke feels strong and my mind is as clear as the water. I'm still feeling apprehensive and find myself wondering how I know that I'm nervous. Who is it noticing my nervousness? The butterflies in my stomach, my fretful mind, these are just things I'm experiencing, in the same way as I experience the sensation of cool water around my torso or the mild pain in my left shoulder. I'm not the butterflies. I'm not the anxiety. I'm not the shoulder pain. I'm simply noticing those things. Swimming in the dark seems to be giving me distance to let go of some anchors. It's liberating. And then it's light.

The lake is absolutely stunning. Breathtaking. The water is so clear, you can always see the bed. And turning to breathe is a treat, every single time. Right, the shoreline. Left, the lake, the mountains beyond, and the blood orange sun beginning to rise behind them. Swimming in Lake Tahoe during the sunrise is one of the most magical experiences of my life. The hours pass quickly. Somehow five have gone by as I reach the bear-proof box of goodies I've left myself on the shore.

There's a massive Whole Foods over the road from our lakeside lodge and last night I bought much of the store in anticipation of two long swims. I'm shivering a little as, with holidaying families looking on, I exit the water on unsteady legs and begin inhaling food. Within minutes I've polished off all of today's supply of bars, nuts, fruit and energy drinks – as well as much of tomorrow's. I sense a few people are building up to start asking questions and much as I'd love to tell them what I'm doing, I realise I'm on the clock. I close the box and dive straight back in the lake. It's warmer in the water than out and I have three more hours' steady swimming until I can call it a day.

Those three hours prove pretty easy. The morning clouds over and the visibility comes and goes, as does my mojo. Occasionally I allow my brain to drift to how much longer a Channel swim will be, and how much wavier, and how much colder, and I panic. But most of the time I'm content to put one arm in front of the other in this beautiful lake and wait out the eight hours. As the writer Devin Kelly puts it, there is a sense, while doing something physically hard for a long time, 'of being as far along the edge of yourself as possible.'

That's the point of all of this really. All these silly challenges I set myself… I love that sense of pushing my boundaries. When I think I might be biting off more than I can chew, it feels like I'm sucking all the juice out of this one short life we're blessed to be given.

Just after noon, I'm back in our rented lodge feeling very pleased with myself. I've just swum twice as long as ever before – the day after running a hilly marathon and two days after the epic Alcatraz swim. I'm on a high for the rest of Monday. We embark on a beautiful family hike, glimpsing the lake unfold below us as we climb the surrounding mountains. Then return to the shores and hire a jet ski. Squeeze the throttle and marvel at how quickly you can power down a distance that took hours to swim.

All the while I'm excited to get back in the water tomorrow morning, especially now I know what I'm doing. I feel like I've become some kind of aquatic Duracell bunny. Can I be blamed for the occasional bout of smugness about how well I'm doing? And then Tuesday happens.

Tuesday's long swim is meant to be eight hours, too. It ends up being more like seven and I suffer every second. The magic 'swimming time' thing just never happens. The opposite in fact. Time sags and hours decide to last years. My shoulder complains loudly throughout. By now I'm used to some pain at the start of every swim. It usually fades after around 20 minutes and thereafter rears its head only lightly, briefly, almost tentatively, every half hour or so. But this time the pain just grows and grows until I worry I'm doing myself some proper damage.

I try my old ultra running trick to get rid of pain. The theory goes as follows (and it's my theory by the way, nothing based on anything medical, so buyer beware, though it does work for me): right, so let's say you knee hurts too much to run on. Back in the hunter-gathering days, back when we were persistence hunters who chased down our prey across the African savannah, you couldn't simply put your feet up and rest until your knee recovered, because you'd either be eaten or starve to death. So you'd run through pain and your body would find a way of healing you – literally 'on the run'.

My method of getting rid of pain is to do the opposite of ignoring it. Concentrate on nothing but the pain. Let the pain have the freedom of your mind. Let it flourish. Because there's only a limited amount of information the nerves can send up to the brain and eventually they'll simply be overloaded and give up. At which point, the pain goes from 100 to zero in a heartbeat. Like I say, it really does work for me.

But it doesn't really work during this swim. I'm constantly aware of the nagging burn in my left shoulder as I slowly grind out the two hours in darkness. I'm hoping my mood will improve and my energy will return when it gets light. Neither happens. I'm in a right state when I get back to the bear-proof box. The food defibrillating me is my final hope. Doesn't happen either.

And so the minutes tick by. Sluggishly. Grimly. My shoulder pain runs riot. It mushrooms from nagging to excruciating. I keep reminding myself of the Special Forces mantra: train hard; fight easy. It takes all my determination to keep going, until finally my will-power runs out with an hour to go.

Back at the lodge, Caroline is concerned. I remind her that this will stand me in good stead. I've spent 15 of the past 30 hours in the water. I've done all this training to make sure the Channel swim goes all right. Which turns out not to be a good idea, because the Channel swim does not go all right.

23

Swimming Around

About a year before I was due to swim the Channel, I had been to visit the legendary Sally Minty-Gravett in Jersey and we had a delightful chat over a cup of tea in her front room. Most of that made it into the Swimming Sally chapter, but not this bit:

> 'I booked my two-way for 2014, never even got to Dover because the weather was so bad. In 2015 we went to Dover and waited for two weeks, didn't get my swim done. And then 2016 was my year when I got my two-way done.'

I felt this bit was just a little too mundane. After all, who wants to hear about Channel swims not happening? Move along, nothing to see here. They don't call it the Dover-coaster for nothing.

I was number three on the 10 to 15 September spring tide with well-respected pilot Mike Oram. I never got to meet him. I never got to swim.

Well, nobody got to swim the Channel that week. There's an online link to the GPS location of all the registered boats. I spent the days refreshing that link obsessively and all the boats stayed forlornly moored in Kent.

In all honestly, I'd have struggled to swim anyway. The shoulder which started hurting in Lake Tahoe never stopped hurting. Every stroke with my left arm seemed to exacerbate the pain. Anything over an hour had become excruciating, so no long swims for a month leading up to my tide. I was trying to find the positives, persuading myself that much less swimming – therefore far fewer calories burned – was a win-win; both resting my shoulder and allowing my body to put on that much-needed layer of brown fat to cope with the cold.

Then at the last minute, unusually for me, I took expert advice from both Sally and Mike, and postponed. Literally on the eve of my tide. I'd been grappling with telling the truth about my shoulder, but was determined to tough it out. I didn't much care what state the shoulder would be in afterwards, if only to have a crack at swimming to the Cap. It was only when I finally came clean that I realised the risk I'd have been putting myself and others through.

Mike:

> 'Shoulder injuries in swimming are a serious problem. They take time to recover from and can lead to all sorts of long-term damage.'

Sally:

> 'It's the right decision believe me. You would do irreparable damage to your shoulder swimming for up to 15 hours.'

Crap weather and a crappy shoulder. It seems the Channel wasn't meant to be. I remembered those words of Sally's which initially I'd taken no notice of:

> 'Never even got to Dover because the weather was so bad... Went to Dover and waited for two weeks. Didn't get my swim done.'

I also remembered what had happened to Will Ellis the previous month. His Channel attempt was planned for mid-August. He was given a solid green light for Monday 11 August and put all the many moving parts in place: childcare, family, friends, WhatsApp group, donation link, flights from Jersey for his crew (Sally). He was practically on the A20 on the outskirts of Dover when he was stood down until September due to the weather. Barely a week later there was a last-minute window and he grabbed it. So just before 8am on Sunday 18 August he finally set off on what would turn into a rough – and rather epic – successful crossing.

I wasn't so lucky. It hit me how many people have had to deal with this, both today and over the past century of Channel attempts. Of course, I didn't heed much of Sally's advice and to be completely honest I hadn't put on nearly enough fat. In all probability I would have been pulled hypothermic from the water with a shoulder on fire. But still…

I generally enjoy being haphazard: doing things my way, preparing by barely preparing, battling through (ignoring) bureaucracy, being the last-minute Charlie. I believe that being fit enough – and mentally strong enough – will see me through. And for the Channel, I'd done a thousand per cent more preparation than ever before. I'd been through the required medical, put together a team to support me on the boat (thank you Marlene, thank you James, thank you Caroline).

I'd even filled in all the forms and gone as far as booking an Airbnb near Dover for the week of the swim, only to cancel it when I belatedly realised we live just a couple of hours' drive away and could wait for the call at home. But the Channel requires another level of preparation altogether, along with a level of humility to understand that things are more than likely not to work out how you want them to – whether or not that's your fault.

The disappointment felt like a mini bereavement. Training really hard for something which simply doesn't take place was a new experience and very unpleasant. For days I carried a hole in my stomach and a cloud above my head. I was generally tetchy, even slightly sulky. I tried to show a stoic face to friends and family, making a joke of it, but I suspect everyone saw through me. Even the sound of a tap, a shower, a loo flushing… felt like water was mocking me. I couldn't even bear to look at the Thames as I jogged along the towpath. I knew there was growth here somewhere, but was struggling to find it.

I tried to run my way out of the funk, but it didn't work. I started running with a 20 kilogram weighted vest, just to take my mind off my disappointment. It worked, but only up to a point. In fact, right up to the point I injured my hip by trying too much too soon. I missed swimming, but I was simultaneously cross with swimming, so stayed away from the pools, rivers, lakes and lidos. I didn't even want to see the sea, let alone swim in it.

After a couple of weeks of this grown-up petulance, out of the blue I received an email from my friend Nick. We met seven years previously during a 50-mile running race in the West Country and kept in touch. I hadn't heard from him for months when, in late September, the following landed in my inbox:

'Hey Vassos. How are you? Seen your Channel post. I've not been up to speed and obviously this is disappointing, but just wanted to say that I think this is huge – just the getting yourself ready to go! Appreciate more than a formality to actually do it, but you must have learnt so much and significantly adapted your fitness etc.

'How was the mental bit for you? Of being ready to walk into the sea with the belief you can just keep swimming out and out and out.. until you reach France? Crazy concept. Did you have to work on it? It feels a bit ultimate mentally to me. I get twitchy 100 metres off shore. Think I'm getting better. With family in lakes this year I tried to just swim to the middle of a few nice, quiet lakes and tarns on my own. Beautiful thing to do, but a real mental battle/very twitchy. Hoping I'll flick a switch one day.

'Anyway just wanted to say that's amazing! Well done! I'd expect no less of you, of course, but glad to know you're going to try again next year! All the very best, Nick'

Well, I needed some perspective and Nick started providing it. The fact is, I've enjoyed what it's taken to get to a place where I can even consider swimming the Channel. It's been both fascinating and rewarding – a wonderful journey and I genuinely wouldn't swap any of it. Who'd have thought such a committed runner could fall head over heels in love with swimming?

But that thing Nick mentions about 'flicking the mental switch' to be comfortable swimming out to sea more than 100 metres from shore... He assumes I've managed to conquer that fear. He's 100% wrong about that. Still terrified and reckon I always will be. Then again, the fear only adds to the allure. If it's worth having it doesn't come easy and if it comes easy it usually isn't worth having.

These days Nick tends to enter events with his inspirational daughter Eve, who has a visual impairment. When he sent that email, he and Eve had just raised thousands of pounds for Guide Dogs walking 50 miles together in Devon and Cornwall at the Long-Distance Walking Association's 'Potter Round the Otter' event. I belatedly started to get over myself.

Much as many of us take our eyesight for granted. We also take our ability to swim for granted. We live on an island; water is in our DNA. Swimming seems like a life skill we should all possess. I remembered being at the Henley Swim Festival and meeting a wonderful charity who teach disadvantaged kids to do exactly that. Swim Tayka was founded by a Channel swimmer, Bryan Avery, who visited South America shortly after his successful solo crossing:

'I went out to Lake Titicaca in Peru and found there was no support for the children to teach them to swim. They had no swimming instructors to do it. So I then searched around the world for an organisation that might be able to support them and there wasn't one. That's why Swim Tayka was born.

'*Tayka* – pronounced Tie-Car – means mother in Aymara, the local language. So Swim Mother. We started to reach out to other organisations looking after vulnerable or less fortunate children in low resource environments.

'For instance there's the El Comedor Soup Kitchen where the local women go and of course they bring their children. We collect the kids from that location, take them on a local bus to a local swimming pool and teach them to swim. Swim Tayka basically pays for all that, providing tens of thousands of children with free swimming lessons and transportation.

'And now we've got programmes not only in Peru, but Brazil, Uganda, Bali, Mozambique, Tanzania, Jamaica. If we can get more swimming instructors out to these locations, they would see that these children actually want to learn to swim, as opposed to being told they need to learn. Also, the sheer joy in their faces while they're doing it.

'I remember one of the first years we did it, we had a child who was really angry, used to bite and scratch people. And when we set the swimming programme going, you could see he really wanted to go in the pool, but he would not let go of the handle rails. And after a week and a half, one of the volunteers managed to support him to be able to come off the handle rails, to float, to lie in the pool. And from that point onwards, he was a totally different child. He'd finally given some trust to somebody else – just because he had such a big desire to learn to swim.'

In 2021 the UN General Assembly declared 25 July to be annual Drowning Prevention Day. And two years later passed a resolution requesting member states implement drowning prevention programmes. Swim Tayka are at the forefront of that. Who knows how many lives the charity has saved. It's obviously difficult to quantify, but the sad fact is there are still approximately 42 drowning deaths per hour. Every hour. Swimming is the only sport that can save your life. We should all be able to swim.

And we should all be able to swim safely. In the UK our water, this wonderful life force of ours, is being pumped through with sewage. Our seas, rivers and lakes are being bombarded by unprecedented and unforgivable pollution, mainly from the big water companies. At the time of writing, Thames Water is trying to muscle through a plan to extract millions of gallons of clean water from the river in west London and replace it with sewage. It would be funny if it wasn't so appalling.

The swimmers are fighting back. It's great to be part of the fight. In November 2024 tens of thousands of us descended on Westminster from all corners of the UK to March for Clean Water. People brought placards, celebrities made speeches, families dressed as giant poos. All to make the very reasonable demand that the government stop the poisoning of Britain's waters.

It was the coming together of hundreds of local action groups, from Whitstable to Windermere. I'm also part of the Save Our Lands and River group in Teddington, which is trying to force Thames Water to abandon its horrific plan to build a so-called extraction plant which would replace the river water we swim in with sewage.

A week after Nick's email arrived in my inbox, I find myself defiantly stripping off beside a sign saying 'No swimming' on the shore of a reservoir in the Peak District. I pull on swimming cap and goggles, and slip into the inviting waters. My body takes a minute or so to adjust to the sudden temperature change. As soon as it does, I set off towards the centre with a confident front crawl. My first swim since the disappointment of not attempting the Channel. It hits me like that rush of heat when you step out of the plane on holiday. I love this!

Years ago, at college, in our circle of friends, was a supremely talented badminton player from Jakarta. Michelle taught us a way of saying 'no' in her native Indonesian. *Belum*. It means 'not yet'. I love how there's such optimism and opportunity wrapped up in a supposed negative.

Have you completed your dissertation, Michelle? *Belum*. Do you know how to juggle? Do you speak Spanish? *Belum*. *Belum*.

Have you swum the Channel? *Belum*.

So while the ultimate challenge still eludes me, it's been a delight to delve under the bonnet of open water swimming. The inspiring people I've got to talk to, the communities, the heroism, the stories. I've also got to do an awful lot of swimming, the biggest treat of all.

These days I can't pass a big body of water without wanting to dive in, but I've come to understand that open water swimming is more than just a physical activity. It's a metaphor for life – sometimes chaotic, always unpredictable and ultimately liberating. Every day the world changes us and swimming brings us back to where we come from. It often demands us to dive headfirst into discomfort, to find humour in the struggles and to embrace our inner dolphin, even when we feel more like a soggy sock.

APPENDIX

Marathon swimming rules… Here we go. Both simple and a little complicated. This is from the Marathon Swimmers' Federation (MSF). You need to understand the spirit of all this, before diving into the rules themselves, because the rules are guided by the traditions and spirit of unassisted marathon swimming:

'Marathon swimmers embrace the challenge of crossing wild, open bodies of water with minimal assistance beyond their own physical strength and mental fortitude. There are ways to make the sport easier, but marathon swimmers consciously eschew them.

'Marathon swimmers take pride that their achievements can be meaningfully compared to the achievements of previous generations, because the standard equipment of the sport has not changed significantly since 1875 (when Matthew Webb became the first person to successfully swim the English Channel).

'The declared swim rules must be read aloud by the observer in the presence of the swimmer and all support personnel before the swim begins.

'Start and finish: The swim begins when the swimmer enters the water from a natural shore. If geographic obstacles (e.g. cliffs) prevent the swimmer from clearing the water at the start, the swimmer may begin the swim by touching and releasing from part of the natural shore (e.g. cliff face).

'The swim finishes when the swimmer clears the water on a natural shore, beyond which there is no navigable water. If geographic obstacles prevent the swimmer from clearing the water at the finish, the swimmer may finish by touching part of the natural shore.

'Physical contact: The swimmer may not make intentional supportive contact with any vessel, object, or support personnel at any time during the swim.

'Standard equipment: The swimmer may wear a single textile swimsuit with standard coverage, one latex or silicone cap, goggles, ear plugs, nose clips, and may grease the body. The swimmer may not use any additional equipment that benefits speed, buoyancy, endurance, or heat retention.

'Drafting: The swimmer may not intentionally draft behind any escort vessel or support swimmer. The swimmer may swim alongside an escort vessel, but may not intentionally position him or herself inside the vessel's bow and displacement waves, except while feeding.

'Support swimmers: A support swimmer (or swimmers) may accompany the solo swimmer for a limited duration. Multiple support swims are allowed, but should not occur consecutively. The MSF recommends a maximum of one hour per support swim and a minimum of one hour between support swims.

'The support swimmer may not intentionally touch the solo swimmer and must position him or herself at least slightly behind the solo swimmer.

'Authority on the escort vessel: The observer is responsible for documenting the facts of the swim, interpreting the swim rules, and keeping the official time.

'The pilot of the escort vessel (or lead pilot, if there are multiple vessels) is the ultimate authority in all other matters. The pilot may cancel the swim at any time, for any reason, including, but not limited to, concerns for the safety of the swimmer or support personnel. The pilot is responsible for following all relevant local maritime regulations.

'Responsible environmental stewardship: Everyone involved in the swim attempt – swimmer, observer, support personnel, and escort boat personnel – must treat the environment respectfully and prevent avoidable harm to marine wildlife and ecosystems.

'Continuance of the spirit of marathon swimming: If any issue regarding swim conduct arises that the swim rules do not clearly address, the swimmer should act – and the observer should judge – in accordance with the spirit of unassisted marathon swimming.'

ACKNOWLEDGEMENTS

My friend Lisa works in publishing and collects acknowledgements like Prufrock's coffee spoons. Well, Lisa, this is a big one. The combined brains of my family, Bloomsbury, and the millions listening to Virgin Radio struggled to come up with a suitable title for this book. And just as we were going to have to settle for something pretty average, I mentioned the dilemma to Lisa over lunch in Whitstable. She instantly suggested *Swimmingly*. It's positive, apt and doesn't take itself too seriously; perfect. (I shudder to admit the other contenders, *Running Water, Waterproof, Let the River Run, The High is Tide*... thank goodness for Lisa!)

The swimming community is genuinely welcoming and wonderful. I can't express how grateful I am to everyone who helped along the way, and continues to do so. And of course to the people who enthusiastically agreed to an interview: in order of appearance, Paul Parrish, Ray Gibbs, Marlene Lawrence, Simon Griffiths, Calum Hudson, Keri-Anne Payne, Craig Foster, Sally Minty-Gravett, Alison Macmillan, Julie Bradshaw, Sean Conway, Duncan Goodhew, Rich Roll, Lynne Cox, Will Watt, David Walliams, Lewis Pugh, Will Ellis, Mark Fox, Diana Nyad, Ed Acteson and Bryan Avery. You're all amazing swimmers, and joyful humans. And thanks to Patrick McKeown, the world expert on breathing.

Bloomsbury are a privilege to work with. Thank you especially to Charlotte for your inspiration and friendship, and Sarah for your patience and expertise. Also big thanks to the fantastic Katherine and Cathleen in publicity, Lizzy and

Xanthe in marketing, Julian and his sales team and audiobook Ashleigh. Plus a shoutout to Neil Stevens for another fabulous cover design, our third together.

My smashing family do put up with a lot, particularly when I'm mid-obsession. Training for a solo Channel swim takes up many hours at weekends and during fancy holidays to Mauritius and the USA. Thank you for bearing with me, and pretending to be interested in the latest long swim. I've fallen madly in love with swimming (you may have noticed), but Caroline, Emily, Matthew, Mary, I love you ever so much more.

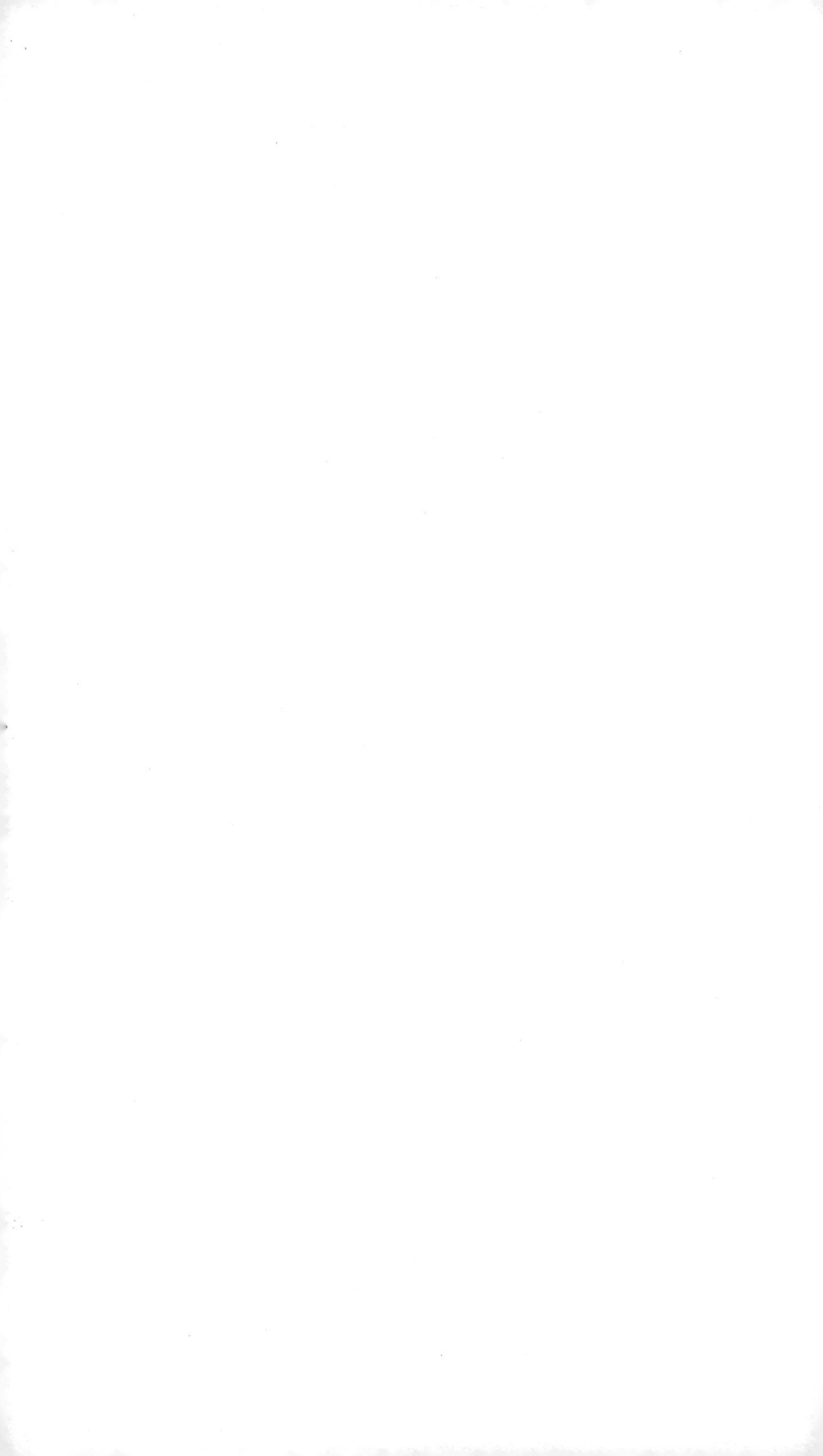